# Common Psychiatric Emergencies

GRAEME McGRATH MA, DPhil, MRCPsych
*Lecturer in Psychiatry*
*Department of Psychiatry, University Hospital of South Manchester*

MALCOLM BOWKER PhD MRCPsych
*Consultant Psychiatrist*
*Samuel Falk Centre, Birch Hill Hospital, Rochdale*

**WRIGHT**
Bristol
1987

© **IOP Publishing Limited.** 1987

*Published under the Wright imprint by*
IOP Publishing Limited
Techno House, Redcliffe Way, Bristol BS1 6NX.

*British Library Cataloguing in Publication Data*

McGrath, Graeme
    Common psychiatric emergencies.
    1.      Psychiatric emergencies
    I.     Title    II. Bowker, Malcolm
    616.89′025    RC480.6

ISBN 0 7236 0806 1

*Typeset by*
Severntype Repro Services Ltd,
Market Street, Wotton-under-Edge, Glos.

*Printed in Great Britain by*
The Bath Press,
Lower Bristol Road, Bath BA2 3BL.

# Preface

It is common for members of all the caring professions to be faced with having to deal with psychiatric problems in those who turn to them for help. Despite this, many problems involving psychological distress or disturbance arouse feelings of anxiety, distress or hostility in those who could provide help. Psychiatry, no less than any other branch of medicine, is a practical pursuit. The aim of this book is to provide practical guidelines for those who find themselves responsible for managing acute psychiatric disturbance.

Although aimed primarily at hospital workers—house officers, casualty officers, junior psychiatrists in training, nurses and other paramedical staff—we hope that the advice contained will be useful to those outside the hospital, including general practitioners, counsellors, police, the clergy and others who may meet such problems as part of their professional life. We make no apology for adopting a conventional clinically-based schema for the areas covered by specific chapters.

The wish to understand individuals in a complete sense (from each of the physical, psychological and social perspectives) has always been an essential component of good medical practice. The individual professional's temperament will to a great extent determine his stance on such issues, but neglect of any of these overlapping areas of understanding will lead to inadequate assessment and treatment. The aim of medical practice is to assist the 'patient' towards a state of increased autonomy, whether the restricting factor be a fractured femur or a psychiatric illness. The doctor who triumphantly produces movement in an apparently paralysed limb by applying painful pressure or excess heat to the skin (thus 'demonstrating' that the patient is 'malingering') is not practising medicine. He may in fact be perpetuating a way of maladaptive coping with emotional problems which (with a little more thought and patience) could have been altered in a constructive way. We are in broad agreement with Murphy and Guze (1960) that terms such as manipulative and malingering are pejorative and value-laden unless used in clearly defined contexts and are best abandoned for a more neutral description of actual *behaviour* wherever possible.

If the duty doctor in the psychiatric unit or casualty department can develop the capacity to approach the 'awkward', 'attention-seeking' 'psychiatric' patient with the mental set that, however unusual, irritating or threatening a behaviour might seem, in most instances resolution of the problem can be based on understanding and agreement, he will derive more professional satisfaction from the encounter.

The aim of this book therefore is to help in a practical way those professionals who are faced with common psychiatric problems as part of their working routine. This book will not replace more formal psychiatric texts (*see* suggested further reading) but we hope it will complement them, providing a ready source of reference at times when the more leisurely business of full psychiatric assessment is not appropriate.

G. McG.
M.B.

# Contents

# Introduction

Transient emotional disturbance with symptoms of anxiety, depression, elation or anger is a familiar phenomenon and can usually be understood by those who know the individual concerned. *Psychiatric* symptoms—which include disturbances of perception, thinking and consciousness as well as of mood—do not necessarily imply morbidity. The concept of 'illness' is imprecise in both general medicine and psychiatry (not just in the latter as is sometimes implied). Part A of this book deals with approaches to emergency presentations of psychiatric disorder including assessment of patients with psychiatric symptoms, the language of psychiatry, questions of morbidity and illness and the 'medical model' of psychiatric illness. Part A also presents a simplified diagnostic classification of psychiatric illness, covers general principles of emergency management, and ends with a discussion of problems encountered by staff dealing with 'difficult' psychiatric patients, including some of the defensive strategies both patient and staff may adopt in the presence of mental illness or severe emotional distress.

Only a brief outline of the major psychiatric syndromes which can present as emergencies is included (in Part B), following the diagnostic criteria used in the *Diagnostic and Statistical Manual of Mental Disorders* of the American Psychiatric Association (DSM-III).

Where psychiatric symptoms are of morbid intensity, or where there is evidence for delusional or hallucinatory

1

experiences, skill and practice are required to assess and take appropriate action. Part C of the book contains a description of situations posing special difficulties, and in particular suggests practical management strategies for anger, depression and anxiety. Part D considers psychological problems that may occur in general medical and surgical wards.

Part E deals with the management of those individuals who harm themselves either deliberately by self-poisoning or other means, or as a consequence of so-called *substance abuse* (narcotic drugs, alcohol, solvents and glues).

Familiarity with the relatively small number of drugs used for treatment in emergency psychiatry is required and consideration of these, as well as common drugs which can cause psychiatric symptoms, appears in Part F.

The law relating to the compulsory detention and treatment of patients has recently been revised in the Mental Health Act of 1983. The amount of information that a patient may reasonably expect to receive prior to treatment (for example, discussion of alternatives and potential hazards) and the need to consider the capability of the patient to give a valid consent to treatment are increasingly being defined by law. Aspects of the law relevant to emergency psychiatry are discussed in Part G.

It cannot be denied that disturbed behaviour or oddities of conduct are poorly tolerated, not only by the public, but also by staff in general hospitals. This may arise in part from lack of experience in developing the clear, empathic understanding of mental disorder required to approach and treat the mentally distressed in a constructive and confident manner. It is hoped that this book will provide a basis for encouraging both ability and interest in psychological medicine.

Clinical illustrations throughout are drawn from the actual experience of the authors over the past eight years, but we do not suggest they are representative of medical practice whether the incidents described invite censure or praise. The third person *he* is used throughout the text for reasons of economy. *Patient** seems to us to be the most appropriate description from an etymological point of view for those who seek medical help and is used in preference to current alternatives, for example *client.*†

* *Patient* derives from a Latin root meaning to bear and thus has the connotation of 'one who bears or endures suffering'.
† *Client* derives from the Latin word for one dependent upon a patron, and it is precisely this attitude of patronage or 'patronising' that we are keen to avoid.

# Part A
# Approaches to psychiatric disorder

# 1. Approaches to psychiatric illness

Psychiatric illnesses are frequently encountered in medical and other services. Some 10% of patients attending accident and emergency departments are primarily suffering from psychiatric disorders, while psychiatric disturbance can play a part in up to 40% of emergency presentations.

## ASSESSMENT AND RECOGNITION

Psychiatric disorder presenting acutely may be overt (for example, acute psychosis) or hidden by physical symptoms (depression presenting as abdominal pain, alcohol abuse presenting as fits). The disorder and its presentation may be caused by psychological, physical or environmental factors.

When any person requests urgent help from professionals this indicates that a change has occurred which has become intolerable to the patient or to significant others. To the patient or his relatives rapid action often appears essential, but this is rarely the case; precipitate action will only add to anxiety.

## THE FIRST CONTACT WITH THE PATIENT

The patient presenting as an emergency deserves a prompt response to reduce the distress of all concerned. Introducing oneself by name and using the patient's title and surname help to establish an atmosphere of both calm and courtesy, and improve rapport and cooperation between staff and the patient in distress.

Those used to dealing with patients with psychiatric disorders are accustomed to a relatively long period of assessment. In an emergency setting there is an assumption that patients must be assessed and treated quickly, often with only minimal information. Psychiatric problems cannot be dealt with in just a few minutes. It is necessary to allow adequate time, preferably with no interruptions, to make a proper assessment. Patients' and relatives' anxiety will be reduced by explaining how the problem will be assessed, rather than by over-rapid action.

Patients may be confused, suicidal, or suffering from frightening or incomprehensible experiences. They may feel they have little control over aggressive impulses, or impulses to run away. Such patients need to be told exactly what is going on and to have someone with them—if no friend or relative is available then a member of staff should stay while they are waiting for assessment.

## GENERAL RULES FOR APPROACHING PATIENTS

### 1. ESTABLISH EMPATHY

Consider how the patient must feel in the situation he is in. *Empathy* must be clearly distinguished from sympathy, which is too often based on identifying closely with the patient ('I felt that way too when my father died').

### 2. TELL THE PATIENT WHAT YOU THINK

The success of the attempt to understand the patient should be tested. This can be done using phrases such as 'it sounds as if you feel pretty hopeless at the moment' if the patient seems depressed. Even if the understanding gained is wrong or incomplete, this process shows the patient that there is an honest attempt to understand what he is saying, and thus helps to gain his trust.

### 3. ASK THE PATIENT TO RESPOND TO WHAT YOU THINK

The patient should be asked directly if what the interviewer thinks is correct, and if he has anything to add. Non-verbal cues can also indicate correct understanding—for example, increased eye contact or signs of relief or relaxation.

## THE LANGUAGE OF PSYCHIATRY

### 1. THE CONCEPT OF ILLNESS

Illness as a concept is imprecise in both general medicine and psychiatry, not just the latter as is sometimes implied. Once illness is recognised this represents the point at which further investigation, pursuit of diagnosis and treatment may be initiated. A *diagnosis* is the concept of a particular illness—recognised clinically from the history of the illness, including symptoms, and physical examination, supported by special investigations. The illness has a definable onset, progress and resolution, modified in an understandable way by factors peculiar to the individual. If part of the body has been identified as the source of the pathology, and the nature of the lesion demonstrated, the diagnosis may be defined directly in pathological terms. The term 'ill' or 'sick' may be used only if there are morbid symptoms, or (if symptom free) the individual is recognised to be at serious risk of future disability.

Similar diagnostic precision in psychiatry is limited to the so-called organic syndromes (q.v.). Ideally a diagnosis of mental disorder is defined by a statement describing the form of mental dysfunction (e.g. disorder of thought characterised by paraphrasia and neologisms) and other behaviour arising from disturbance of mental function (e.g. verbal responses to apparent auditory hallucinations). Although the content of disturbed mental function may be coloured by social and other cultural factors, this diagnosis of mental dysfunction would be independent of particular social or cultural norms. It is best to avoid terms such as *normal* or *abnormal* as there is no direct link between these concepts and ideas of dysfunction and morbidity.

## 2. THE MEDICAL MODEL

It is beyond dispute that physical insult to the brain, including direct damage, electrical stimulation and the effects of various drugs, can profoundly disturb mental function. It is also common experience to suffer changes of mood in response to various illnesses or medical conditions. The medical component in the study of mental disorders is therefore self-evident. In those mental conditions where biochemical or subtle neuronal disturbance may be implicated (severe depressive and schizophrenic illnesses) there is justified medical interest.

Where problems are thought to arise predominantly from psychological deficiencies or trauma in early life (to over-simplify one theory of the origin of neuroses and personality disorders) the use of the 'medical model' may be questioned. In abbreviated form the argument is that a medical condition does not exist without demonstrable pathology; in addition it may be proposed that medical management in general excludes psychosocial factors both in assessment and treatment. Much has been written on this topic and some references are included in the bibliography. Most psychiatrists take an eclectic approach using counselling, problem solving and other psychological techniques combined with the prescription of drugs and other 'physical' treatment where appropriate. Most would subscribe to the current 'holistic' view that good medical practice includes consideration of the physical, psychological and social aspects of a patient's symptoms or problems.

## 3. PSYCHOLOGICAL TECHNIQUES AND ASSESSMENT

Despite the many named treatments now described in textbooks of psychiatry or practical psychology (behaviour therapy, psychosexual counselling, cognitive therapy, various forms of psychotherapy, etc.), these are not new methods of influencing behaviour. Most psychologically aware individuals will recognise within the methods elements common to the everyday way in which humans try to modify their own and others' behaviour. Psychologists and psychiatrists have simply examined and systematised these unstructured practices into strategies useful in clinical practice, and at the same time developed theoretical models and methods of assessment. Only very few of these relate specifically to emergency psychiatry; for example, rating scales for suicidal intent are available. Psychological assessment will not demonstrate deficits in behaviour that would not be apparent from careful observation of the patient's responses over a period of time. Every doctor should be capable of performing a mental state examination, particularly in order to detect features of organic illness, and of recording the patient's *behaviour* in a way that avoids precipitate speculation and judgement of his assumed motives.

## ASSESSMENT—OBJECTIVITY AND DETACHMENT

Objectivity is not the same as detachment, which is often an attempt by professionals to avoid situations they find difficult or distressing. This failure of empathy is expressed in phrases such as 'pull yourself together' or by stereotyping ('Another overdose—they're just a waste of time'). Such responses cause patients to be uncooperative with assessment and treatment and cause unnecessary suffering to patients and their families. Expressing your understanding of the patient objectively in terms of a general formulation (for example, in terms of medical or psychiatric diagnosis, or psychosocial problems) provides an alternative explanation of the patient's problems, which may point the way to further investigation and management.

In an assessment interview any topic of concern to the patient may be talked about, however far it may seem from the presenting complaint ('It sounds as though you've not been coping at work so well recently—would you like to tell me a bit more about that?'). When dealing with strong emotions it must be made clear that talking is seen as better than acting ('People quite often feel so angry they'd like to hit someone, but I guess it's important to avoid that. What's been getting you so uptight?'). Talking by itself can be therapeutic. This most commonly occurs when the patient can express previously bottled-up ideas or emotions.

## THE EMERGENCY PSYCHIATRIC INTERVIEW

### 1. INTERVIEW STRUCTURE

An emergency interview follows a standard structure. Examination of the mental state should continue throughout the interview. More formal tests of intellectual and cognitive functioning should be performed last. Essential information may need to be elicited quickly and accurately. *Table* 1.1. outlines the minimum information necessary for adequate assessment.

### 2. UNDERSTANDING THE PRESENTATION

The interview should not only provide the interviewer with information for making a formal diagnosis, but must also provide an answer to the question: Why is *this* patient presenting in *this way* at *this time?* The story elicited must make sense in terms of general psychiatric or medical knowledge and in terms of relevant psychological and social factors. If it does not then some important facts are missing.

Even with the most careful interviewing some patients, especially confused, demented or very suspicious or paranoid patients, will be unable or unwilling to give a coherent history. In many cases the mental state examination gives important clues to the nature of the patient's problems (e.g. disorientation, suspiciousness or hostility). Some patients may not wish, or be able, to ask directly for what they want

*Table* 1.1  ASSESSMENT OF PATIENTS WITH SUSPECTED PSYCHIATRIC ILLNESS

Chief complaint
History of present complaint
Past history
  —Psychiatric
  —Family psychiatric
  — Medical
  —Personal
  —Alcohol and drug use
Demographic data and current social situation
Mental status examination
  —Appearance and behaviour
  —Speech
  —Affect and mood
  —Thought
  —Perceptual disturbances
  —Sensorium and cognitive functions
  —Judgement and insight

(the 'hidden agenda') because they feel ashamed, or fear rejection or criticism.

## 3. DISCUSSION WITH THE PATIENT

In most cases it is helpful for the interviewer to discuss his understanding of the problem with the patient. Even confused and psychotic patients will be reassured and more cooperative if they feel they have been listened to and understood. Spelling out the problem also provides a basis for asking the patient more directly what he wants from the emergency service. A direct, non-judgemental approach will often allow the patient to be more forthcoming and help clarify any hidden agenda.

## MENTAL STATE EXAMINATION

As with the physical examination the mental state examination records the interviewer's objective observations of the patient's behaviour, mood, thought, perception and expressed belief during the interview. It represents the *current* state of the patient and should not include historical information.

The main headings under which the mental state examination is traditionally recorded are described briefly below, with some useful questions for eliciting information given in italics (taken from *The Psychiatric Present State Examination*, Wing et al., 1974). A fuller account is given in Appendix 1. In an emergency setting often only the most directly relevant information can be obtained (for example, full cognitive assessment usually need not be performed on a young, fully orientated patient presenting with symptoms of anxiety). Descriptions should be in everyday language and represent an objective assessment. Value-laden phrases such as 'attention seeking' or 'manipulative' should be avoided.

## 1. APPEARANCE AND BEHAVIOUR

A description of *appearance* should include the amount of eye contact and any unusual or idiosyncratic features of dress, grooming, expression, posture or movement.

The description of *behaviour* should include the patient's general attitude and cooperation, as well as the level and quality of motor activity and an indication of the interviewer's rapport with the patient.

## 2. SPEECH AND LANGUAGE

*Speech* is characterised by its rate, volume, form and quality. Content of speech is usually recorded under other headings such as mood, thought or perception.

## 3. MOOD

*Mood* is usually described both in the patient's own words (so-called 'subjective' mood) and in terms of emotions detected by the observer ('objective' mood). Description of mood should include comment on the range and appropriateness of emotional expression.

*Have there been times lately when you have been very anxious or frightened?*
*Do you keep reasonably cheerful or have you been very depressed or low-spirited recently?*

## 4. THOUGHT

The patient's *thought* processes are only accessible to an observer through his words and actions, and so description of thought processes is closely related to the descriptions of talk and behaviour. Assessment includes:

  a. *Form of thought.* Disordered thought may be shown by:
    i.   Circumstantiality
    ii.  Tangentiality
    iii. Flight of ideas
    iv.  Loose associations
    v.   Clang associations

  b. *Thought content*—impoverished, or containing morbid ideas or beliefs or suicidal ideations or intent (q.v.). Morbid thoughts with specific definitions include:
    i.   Ideas of reference
    ii.  Delusions
    iii. Obsessions
    iv.  Phobias

*Can you think clearly or is there any interference with your thoughts?*
*Do your thoughts tend to be muddled or slow?*
*Are you in full control of your thoughts?*
*Can people read your mind? (Is something like telepathy going on?)*
*Do you feel under the control of some force or power other than yourself?*
*Is anyone trying to harm you, e.g. trying to poison you or kill you?*

*Is there anything special about you? Do you have special abilities or powers?*

## 5. PERCEPTUAL DISTURBANCES

*Hallucinations* can occur in all sensory modalities, and are common in psychosis and organic disorders. Other perceptual disturbances include illusions, depersonalisation and derealisation.

*Do you ever hear noises or voices when there is no-one about, and nothing else to explain them?*
*Do you have visions or other unusual experiences?*

## 6. COGNITIVE FUNCTION

This is usually formally tested at the end of the interview, although an assessment of attention, concentration, distractibility and level of consciousness can be made during the interview.

   a. *Orientation* is tested by asking the patient's name, age, date of birth: present place, address and town: the day, date and time.

   b. *Memory*
      i.   Registration is tested by the ability to repeat a series of numbers, or a previously unknown name and address immediately after hearing them.
      ii.   Immediate recall is tested by asking the patient to repeat a complex sentence, or the details of a brief story.
      iii.   Recent memory is tested by asking for recall of a name and address after 5 minutes.
      iv.   Remote memory is tested by accuracy of historical information. Confirmation from an informant other than the patient is required.

c. *Abstract thinking* can be assessed by giving the patient proverbs to interpret.

d. *Calculation* may be tested by asking the patient to serially subtract 7, starting from 100.

e. *Tests of constructional ability* include copying designs, drawing a cube or a bicycle, or putting the hands on a clock face.

### 7. JUDGEMENT AND INSIGHT

*Judgement* is a measure of the patient's ability to see the consequences of his actions. *Insight* refers to the patient's understanding of his illness.

## MORBIDITY

*Psychiatric symptoms* including disturbances of consciousness, mood, perception and thinking can arise from a multitude of conditions and their presence (including delusions and hallucinations) does not necessarily imply morbidity. All such phenomena may be encountered in healthy individuals under certain circumstances: the morbid nature of symptoms, alone or in combination, is a matter of judgement. There is no satisfactory definition of 'mental health'. The point at which health is considered to merge into 'sickness' is arbitrarily defined by those (including the patient) primarily concerned with the disturbance or distress caused by symptoms. Sickness may go unrecognised.

## DIAGNOSIS

The first task of the doctor presented with a mental disorder in a patient is to identify any physical (also termed organic) condition such as infection, drug abuse or head injury which may be implicated as a sole or contributory cause of the disorder (organic brain syndromes—q.v.).

This is rarely difficult in practice unless the patient is aggressive or seriously disturbed, making adequate history taking and examination impossible. It is important not to jump to premature conclusions in such cases. It can never be assumed that an individual smelling of alcohol and apparently intoxicated is suffering from the effects of alcohol alone. There may be serious systemic illness, other drugs involved or head injury. 'Smells of whisky; slurred speech; ataxia' is a preferable clinical description to 'intoxicated'—the latter representing a diagnostic judgement usually unsupported by the necessary investigations.

Disturbed behaviour or oddities of conduct may be poorly tolerated not only by the public, but also by doctors and other health service staff. This attitude may arise in part from a lack of confidence in dealing with psychiatric disorder, including the lack of a suitable vocabulary for understanding and describing psychiatric disorder. It is not suggested that non-psychiatric doctors and paramedical staff, particularly in the pressured atmosphere of busy accident and emergency departments or acute admission wards, need be concerned with the minute detail of psychiatric syndromes, but access to a copy of the *Diagnostic and Statistical Manual of Mental Disorders* (DSM-III) of the American Psychiatric Association is recommended, as this offers the vocabulary and concepts that will raise competence in describing and classifying psychiatric disorder—an important step in guiding management. There is extensive overlap between the diagnostic systems of DMS-III and that contained in the *Manual of the International Statistical Classification of Diseases, Injuries and Cause of Death* (ICD-9).

## FRANK'S CLASSIFICATION

Frank (1979) groups mental disorders into categories which provide a simplified classification of mental disorder for professionals requiring a readily remembered framework for emergency and crisis intervention strategies.

## 1. PATIENTS WITH PSYCHOTIC ILLNESS

*Psychosis:* A mental disorder in which impairment of mental function has developed to a degree that interferes grossly with insight, ability to meet ordinary demands of life or to maintain adequate contact with reality. It is not an exact or well-defined term (ICD-9).

This category includes severe depression, mania and acute schizophrenia. Delerium and dementia are included, and severe reactions to stress (following bereavement or natural disaster for instance) may produce a reactive mental state fulfilling the above definition. In severe cases of anorexia nervosa the disturbance of perception, lack of concern for gross emaciation and fear of fatness may justifiably be thought of as psychotic phenomena.

It is usually not possible to arrive at a diagnosis, nor appropriate to discuss possible diagnosis with the patient or relatives until there has been adequate time for observation under psychiatric care. Occasionally lack of insight or dangerous behaviour may necessitate recommending that the patient be compulsorily detained in hospital. All these issues are discussed later in this book.

The interviewer may have difficulty empathising with the patient's experiences, especially when there is disorder of thought or language. Inexperienced interviewers may misinterpret psychotic thinking as awkwardness, neurotic introspection or the oddities of verbal 'game playing'.

## 2. PATIENTS WITH NEUROTIC ILLNESS

The term *neurotic* has currency as a pejorative description, and while useful in considering a practical simplified classification of mental disorders, is a term best avoided when writing or speaking about individual patients. In DSM–III use of the word neurotic is discouraged and these states are included in the classes of affective, anxiety, somatoform and other disorders.

Frank's definition is succinct:

*Neurotic* people are those who suffer from persistent faulty strategies for dealing with the vicissitudes of life, based presumably on important early experiences that were either damaging or lacking, thereby distorting the processes of maturation and learning.

This may be combined with the ICD–9 definition:

*Neurotic disorders* are mental disorders without any demonstrable organic basis in which the patient may have considerable insight and has unimpaired reality testing, in that he usually does not confuse his subjective experiences and fantasies with external reality. Behaviour may be greatly affected although usually remaining within socially acceptable limits, but personality is not disorganised. The principle manifestations include excessive anxiety, hysterical symptoms, phobias, obsessional and compulsive symptoms and depression.

Within the range of symptoms associated with neurotic illness a commonly misused term is *hysteria*. This word should be reserved for conversion (paralysis, anaesthesia, etc.) or dissociative (fugue, amnesia, etc.) symptoms. *Histrionic* is the appropriate term for dramatic overreaction, shallow emotionality and suggestibility.

It is important to appreciate that the degree of suffering in neurotic disorders can be as severe as that experienced in psychotic illness, particularly where anxiety, depression or disabling obsessive–compulsive symptoms are present. Healthy appearance and the preservation of general abilities including reasoning can hinder empathy with the struggle that the individual experiences in changing his behaviour. The pejorative use of the word neurotic is some recognition of the persistence of faulty strategies despite all support and help. The lay view might be that the patient lacks the will to alter his behaviour in an apparently simple and common-sense way.

The need for psychiatric admission is less for neurotic disorders, but presentation as an emergency may come after many months of struggle with symptoms and indicate a crisis where brief 'asylum' may be appropriate or an underlying associated stress such as a depressive or other illness.

## 3. PATIENTS WHO ARE 'PSYCHOLOGICALLY SHAKEN'
Frank:
Those who are temporarily overwhelmed by current life stresses such as bereavement. Relatively brief and superficial help usually suffices to restore their emotional equilibrium.

Within this group are those suffering from uncomplicated bereavement and from adjustment disorders. Most people can empathise with these individuals and deal with the need for the sufferer to relate in detail or repetitively an account of their particular trauma. Adjustment reactions may move imperceptibly into major depressive illness or be confused with stress-evoked exacerbations of traits in the personality disordered.

## 4. PATIENTS WHO ARE 'UNRULY'
Frank:
... whose behaviour upsets other people but is attributed to illness rather than wickedness.

This category includes young people with emotional disturbance who truant from school or act in other ways disturbing to parents and others, patients with personality disorders, and substance abusers. 'Unruly' implies deviation from the social norms, including the law.
To what extent can such behaviour be understood in terms of illness? Scientific and philosophical ideas about illness and wickedness, free will and responsibility may differ greatly

from common usage and legal definitions of these terms. It is, however, by the use of such concepts that decisions are taken to help, reject or censure these individuals.

It is generally accepted that anyone experiencing distortions of perception is unlikely to be as competent functionally as when free of such symptoms. In broad terms they are considered to be less 'responsible' for their actions. If someone demonstrates persisting callous disregard for others, impetuous violence or is simply unpleasant then responsibility for their actions tends to be assumed. If 'functional competence' is measured by any testable aspect of mental activity, including its behavioural consequences, then it is difficult to accommodate the view that an individual should be more responsible for morbid lack of feeling than for morbid changes in affect. Indeed many of the characteristics of sociopathic personalities can be viewed as neurotic in form.

It is helpful when presented with someone who is 'difficult', or who is arousing strong negative feelings to adopt a neutral stance. The first task is to respond in such a way that the apparently inevitable negative consequences of the patient's behaviour are minimised. The negative feelings of the interviewer and others are just as inevitable until this stance is adopted, when such responses are likely to abate. These points are covered more fully in Chapter 3.

Earlier in this chapter the point was made that the diagnosis of mental disorder should be independent of any reference to social or cultural norms. Where the expression of cruelty, violence, remorse, or the quality of relations between people are considered, the decision to label a particular behaviour as morbid (which is a criterion for intervention) will again be arbitrary but also less consistent among those with professional opinions because at this level of behaviour there is more intrusion of personal conviction than with the consideration of other psychiatric disorders.

In practical terms, whatever the status of 'unruly'

behaviour within the rubric of 'mental disorder', the individual, his relatives and friends may wish to know what are the possibilities for dealing with the problem, including legal aspects if applicable.

Individuals, often with chronic mental illness, who live a drifting existence, perhaps associated with alcoholism and homelessness, may also attend or be referred to accident and emergency departments (see Chapter 12). A frequent precipitant for seeking help is physical illness and this should receive primary consideration as it may go unrecognised.

In summary, the medical model—primarily a scientific approach—remains the most appropriate and comprehensive available for recognising mental disorder and organising management. The above simplified description of mental disorder and associated behavioural disorders is described to enable the examining doctor to decide fairly early in the interview the category to which the patient most probably belongs. It should then be possible to anticipate requirements in terms of the time required for interview and examination, any immediate measures to reduce distress or disturbance, the need for the presence of relatives, social workers, police or others and whether psychiatric consultation or admission is required.

## EMERGENCY TELEPHONE CALLS

Patients often telephone hospitals and ask to speak to the psychiatrist on duty. Other agencies may also receive telephone calls, and some like the Samaritans are set up specifically for that purpose. Reasons for telephoning include reasonable requests for help or advice such as desperation in a suicidal or depressed patient, questions about medication or side-effects, or a relative calling about problems managing a patient. Some calls may be less reasonable such as the patient who repeatedly takes overdoses reporting how many tablets have been taken this time, or dissatisfied patients with a stream of complaints.

Whatever the purpose of the telephone call it is essential to get the caller's name, address, telephone number and details of current psychiatric treatment if any. If the patient will not give this information, then he should be told that without it no help can be forthcoming. It is a mistake to argue or get involved in a prolonged struggle with such patients. If several polite and reasonable attempts have failed, then the call should be ended after telling the patient so.

In many cases the telephone contact relieves the immediate problem and further contact, if required, can be organised on a routine basis. If the situation is more urgent then the patient should be invited to come to the emergency department or psychiatric department, and if necessary the police or ambulance services can be contacted. The patient should be told that such help has been requested, and may be kept talking until it arrives.

# 2. Emergency interventions

## IMMEDIATE MANAGEMENT

Patients present as emergencies because of acute, distressing and destabilising changes, and the initial response must be towards stabilisation of the patient and his situation. Examples of such unstable situations include agressive or disturbed patients where there is a risk of violence (q.v.); parasuicide (q.v.); intoxication (q.v.); and acute psychosis (q.v.).

It is essential not to overlook medical conditions that can produce abnormal behaviour, speech or perception such as hypertensive and hepatic encephalopathies, drug and alcohol withdrawal, meningitis, encephalitis, poisoning, hypoxia and hypoglycaemia. These may be missed in difficult, abusive or disturbed patients, who may be discharged or referred on prematurely.

The majority of patients presenting as emergencies with psychiatric symptoms are dealt with by the emergency services or other agencies without referral to a phychiatrist. On some occasions psychiatric referral or admission may be necessary, and this is dealt with later.

There are two distinct parts to the management of patients presenting in psychosocial crisis: dealing with the change that has precipitated the current presentation, and negotiating plans for further treatment if necessary.

## NON-SPECIFIC INTERVENTIONS

1. *Assessment* - the process of interviewing a patient or significant others—will often clarify the nature of the crisis for everyone involved, and may be sufficient to allow the patient to regain his lost sense of control, or to delay until more formal intervention can be offered.

2. *Discussion* of personal problems in a *supportive* way plays a large part in resolving a crisis. This theme is developed below in the section on crisis intervention.

3. The provision of *specific information* about the patient's illness, the nature and effect of any treatment or the availability of other support services can correct misapprehensions and reduce anxiety that may be fuelling the crisis.

4. The use of *psychotropic drugs* is rarely indicated in the emergency situation, and medication should not normally be prescribed except by the person who is going to follow the patient up later.

Possible pharmacological interventions include:

— treating depression if this is interfering with a patient's coping abilities;
— restoring sleep if this is acutely disturbed. There is little indication for long-term hyponotic use;
— giving adequate analgesia;
— reducing anxiety—benzodiazepines can be used for *short-term* reduction of handicapping anxiety that persists despite ventilation of problems and adequate provision of information.

Drugs and advice are usually the first tools to be considered by medically qualified helpers. They have a very limited role in the management of psychiatric emergencies, and should only be given for well-defined reasons and then only sparingly.

## CRISIS INTERVENTION TECHNIQUES

Crisis intervention techniques work best in relatively stable people with transitory but severe difficulties. These include deliberate self-harm and other abnormal behavioural responses to social crises, and severe or inappropriate responses to acute stress such as bereavement. However, the general approach to problems will often be of short-term help even in more disturbed or socially disrupted patients, as part of a longer-term treatment strategy. Some patients may require repeated interventions in recurring crises.

A useful summary of crisis intervention techniques can be found in Bancroft (1979). The emphasis in crisis intervention is that even if the patient is suffering from a serious illness, he and his family have a share in the responsibility for coping with their difficulties.

In an emergency the aim is to help the patient define and take control of the crisis, working with his strengths to renew his feelings of competence and mastery. The patient is helped to define the problem, generate new solutions and work towards accomplishing them, and to do this the helper must use a structured, empathic, problem-solving approach.

a. *Reduce anxiety* and emotional arousal that interferes with problem-solving. It is usually possible to do this by patient listening and talking to the patient. Ventilation of powerful suppressed feelings, for example grief or anger, can be a valuable first step when those emotions are appropriate and understandable. Some patients (for example, the acutely psychotic or sociopathic and aggressive) should be encouraged to limit emotional display.

b. *Problem-solving* involves seven stages. These may also help the patient understand the nature of his problem and how it arose:

1. Identify the problem (in practical terms: not 'I can't cope' but 'how can I avoid hitting my baby when I'm feeling so angry?').
2. Propose alternative solutions. The patient should be guided to his own solutions ('I can understand how distressed you are by what's happened. I wonder if you've thought of any ways you might improve things?').

3. Rehearse alternatives until any implications are clear (by asking what the next step might be, how the patient would take it, what might get in the way, who might help, what the outcome might be).
4. Choose the solution that seems most attractive and possible.
5. Define the steps needed to carry it out (these should be broken down into small and manageable steps).
6. Carry out the proposed course of action.
7. Check the result.

Directive advice and hasty reassurance should be avoided, as they rarely help a patient feel more competent or responsible. If the patient is returning for a follow-up appointment then steps 6 and 7 above can be agreed as a task for the patient to work on.

The patient should be helped to realise that he has learnt a general technique for coping with future crises, as well as being helped with the current difficulty.

In many cases it will be appropriate to take over responsibility for the patient and encourage dependency, for example by hospital admission. This is necessary, for example, with acute organic brain syndromes (q.v.) and some acute psychoses (q.v.), but can be an effective part of crisis intervention, giving a brief period of 'intensive care' to patients who have become exhausted or have completely decompensated until their own resources can be mobilised.

## ASSOCIATED SOCIAL OR INTERPERSONAL PROBLEMS—THE MEDICAL SOCIAL WORKER

In many cases symptoms of psychiatric disorder will be associated with social or interpersonal problems that may be causing or exacerbating the psychological symptoms. In such cases, drawing the attention of the medical social work department to the patient and his needs can be of value. As with all professional referrals it is advantageous to contact the social worker personally to discuss the problems and possible interventions.

In general, social workers are skilled and keen to be involved in four main areas of care:

1. Further *assessment of the family*—enquiring into home circumstances, family support and interaction and identifying areas of special need.
2. Helping with *specific practical needs*—patients who are isolated, have physical disabilities or whose caretakers are infirm, for example. Medical social workers liaise with other services and help organise such things as home helps, meals on wheels, family aids, day centres.
3. Helping to *deal with family disturbance*—meeting the family, domiciliary visits, counselling and family intervention.
4. *Dealing with loss*—working with both patient and family. Losses include both bereavement and loss of important aspects of health or functioning.

Many patients who deliberately poison or harm themselves (q.v.) have severe social problems and no psychiatric illness. There is usually pressure for such patients to be discharged within 24 to 36 hours of admission. In such cases duty psychiatrists are often tempted to declare the patient 'not psychiatrically ill' and refer him to the medical social worker. However, because of the special nature of their work, medical social workers deal primarily with patients who have chronic illness, or who remain as in-patients for some time, and have little to offer patients who leave hospital rapidly. In these cases it is essential to speak to the social worker personally *before the patient is discharged* to discuss what can be offered. The social worker might be in the best position to alert the area social services team, for example, but expectations of what medical social wokers can achieve in these situations should not be exaggerated.

## REFERRAL TO A PSYCHIATRIST

In emergency settings contact with psychiatrists should be made directly over the telphone so that the reasons for referral, problems and information available can be clarified. The question the psychiatrist is expected to answer must be clearly defined. Referral must include the patient's name, sex, age, current location, presenting problems, medical and psychiatric diagnoses (if known) and any relevent past history, especially psychiatric (past psychiatric notes may be available that will materially affect assessment and treatment).

To psychiatrists used to dealing with acute distress a problem might not seem urgent, but urgent referrals indicate anxiety in those trying to help the patient. It is best to respond rapidly to such anxiety, even if the intervention with the patient is limited to a brief assessment and arranging follow-up.

*Case example.* The psychiatrist on call was contacted on a Saturday morning by the duty medical officer, who began with the words 'I've got three overdoses here and no beds so I want you to come and get rid of them.' The psychiatrist responded angrily 'by the book' and told the referring doctor that he did not consider these cases to be emergencies. Fortunately both doctors were sufficiently sensible to make contact later that morning and arrange for the patients to be seen that day.

In most cases referral to a psychiatric out-patient clinic is all that is required. Reasons that patients might be referred to psychiatrists as emergencies include:

1. *Deliberate self-harm* and self-poisoning. Referral should not be made until the patient has been cleared as medically fit, and psychiatric assessment is possible (for

example, the patient is not drowsy from the effects of drugs taken).

2. The patient poses a *management problem*, usually because of disturbed or violent behaviour.
3. If the patient *requires admission* for a psychiatric problem, for example if he is actively suicidal or psychotic.
4. If the *psychiatric diagnosis is unclear* and a specialist opinion is requested.
5. If it is considered that *specialist treatment or advice* is required, for example management of the psychiatric features of delirious states.

Direct referral to other agencies, for example social workers or clinical psychologists for anxiety management, can be more acceptable to some patients and their relatives and less stigmatising than referral to a psychiatrist.

## PSYCHIATRIC ADMISSION

In some cases the patient will need to be admitted to a psychiatric unit. When admission is arranged for a patient his family, general practitioner and any other agencies who may be involved should be informed as soon as possible. Liaison with ambulance and other staff must be adequate to ensure safe and uncomplicated transfer of both patient and essential clinical information from the emergency area to the psychiatric ward. Usually the psychiatrist who has accepted the patient will perform these tasks, but it is the responsibility of the person making the original referral to ensure that all arrangements are completed satisfactorily.

# 3. 'Difficult patients' and professional responses

Clinical situations posing special difficulties for staff (e.g. intoxicated, aggressive or homeless patients) are discussed in later sections of this book. This chapter deals with aspects of the presentation of psychiatric problems which may arouse strong negative responses in staff and thus interfere with effective management.

Many professionals find it hard to understand and deal with psychiatric illness and the patient's behaviour may often intensify the response of anxiety or anger. Negative reactions to apparently maladaptive behaviour are made more likely by the nature of emergency work, where there is pressure to assess and solve problems rapidly and effectively. It is easy to blame the patient for the crisis they are in and neglect proper assessment and treatment.

Factors that provoke negative feelings in staff include:

a. the expression of especially intense feelings (fear, pain, psychotic ideas, hopelessness);
b. unpredictability;
c. coerciveness or passivity;
d. repeated presentation in crisis, often with poor compliance with treatment;
e. the lack of other support (homelessness, loneliness).

Understanding the nature of these difficulties, being aware of one's reactions and using appropriate management skills will help to overcome such problems.

Patients who repeatedly present to the emergency department can be particularly frustrating for staff, especially when treatment has little observable effect and compliance is poor. They may have no other support, seem unable to cooperate with ongoing supervision or treatment, or have been repeatedly rejected by their families, general practitioners and other agencies.

Such situations may put staff in the difficult position of having to choose between offering help that is bound to fail and seeing oneself as rejecting a patient in distress. All carers have the desire and need to help others effectively, but factors in the patient, his family and his social environment may produce more profound changes then any treatment. There are practical limits to the responsibility one can accept for aspects of a patient's life that are beyond one's ability to alter.

## NEGATIVE REACTIONS

Recognising, understanding and managing one's own negative reactions is the key to dealing with these difficult situations. Identifying and accepting such reactions in ourselves may not be easy, and conflict with our views of ourselves as caring professionals. It is easier to explain away 'unprofessional' feelings and behaviour, or to blame them on outside circumstances, than to recognise them as valuable clinical information.

Negative feelings include anxiety (varying in intensity from mild unease and uncertainty to panicky feelings of not being able to cope), anger (including feeling bored, fed-up or frustrated) and pessimism (including feelings of personal inadequacy). These feelings may be expressed as irrational thoughts produced more by emotion than logic.

*Case example.* A young woman, a medical student, took an overdose of antidepressants when severely depressed. As she was brought into casualty, drowsy but conscious, she clearly heard the doctor say 'Not another bloody overdose—it's always a waste of time treating them.'

Some patients manage to get others to take their remarks personally ('You really want me not to sleep at all don't you';

'You're the first doctor I've found that offered me any help'). It may be hard not to overreact to patient's insults or threats, often by taking too much personal responsibility for the patient's condition ('If that patient leaves here and kills himself I'll get the blame').

Sometimes staff respond 'unprofessionally' because of more or less conscious prejudice (for example, treating homosexual patients with sexual problems less sympathetically than heterosexual patients), or because the patient's problems reflect their own in some way.

*Case example.* A patient presented as an emergency with severe anxiety, unable to cope at home when his wife was in hospital. The duty psychiatrist, whose own wife had recently been in hospital with an acute and very serious illness, refused the demands for medication and offered an out-patient appointment at an unspecified future time for anxiety management training. The patient left angrily and presented to out-patients some weeks later refusing to see the previous psychiatrist. He had been abusing alcohol and benzodiazepines in the intervening period.

Negative feelings and thoughts can appear as behaviours directed to the patient which hinder effective management, such as arguing, being condescending, insulting him behind his back, not listening to him or discharging him prematurely. Sometimes medication is used inappropriately to get rid of patients, for example giving in to demands for excessive quantities of sedatives.

## WAYS OF COPING WITH POWERFUL FEELINGS

Psychological distress may appear in a number of forms, for example anxiety, depression, shame, guilt, anger or fear. Most individuals wish to experience such distress in as mild a form and for as short a time as possible. Distress may be dealt with in a conscious, rational way (using 'problem-solving' techniques, suppression, or by deliberately distracting oneself). Alternatively individuals may use one of a number of so-called *defence mechanisms* (theoretical unconscious mental processes) in the case of potential distress. These occur essentially outside conscious awareness, and 'defend' the feelings that provoke the anxiety reaching the level of conscious thought.

George Vaillant, in long-term studies of the adjustment of adults to life's problems, correlated relative freedom from mental illness with the use of certain defence mechanisms. A much simplified and abbreviated version of his classification of defence mechanisms is outlined in *Table* 3.1. To this list

*Table* 3.1. EXAMPLES OF PSYCHOLOGICAL DEFENCE MECHANISMS

| Type of defence | Examples | Perceived as |
|---|---|---|
| Immature defences | Passive agression<br>Regression<br>Denial<br>Projection | Misbehaviour |
| Neurotic defences | Dissociation<br>Displacement<br>Intellectualisation | Personal idiosyncracies |
| Mature defences | Altruism<br>Humour<br>Sublimation | Valued characteristics |

might be added prayer and faith, stoicism and fatalism. No classification could capture the wide range and subtle variations of defences employed by all of us. Being aware of and sensitive to such manoeuvres in oneself as well as in others provides a greater understanding of and empathy for the underlying distress behind many forms of apparently maladaptive behaviour. Examples are given below.

*MENTAL HEALTH AND DEFENCE MECHANISMS*
Mental health is difficult to define (see Chapter 1), but if defined as adaptation to life with freedom from psychological

morbidity then a mentally healthy person will employ a wide range of defence mechanisms, with a bias towards more mature defences. Someone whose response to life consisted primarily of denial of reality and acceptance of internal fantasy would be considered a seriously disturbed person whose problems will cause suffering to himself and probably others—these conditions are seen in psychotic illnesses and some of the more severe personality disorders (q.v.).

The use of defence mechanisms can be seen as enabling an individual to cope with information or situations experienced as unbearable. An example would be the patient who has widespread cancer who remains totally unaware of the diagnosis (or even its possibility) even following admission to a hospice in a severely debilitated state (the defence of *denial*).

*Repression* underlies all defences and is the process whereby aspects of experience such as thoughts or feelings are eliminated from conscious awareness.

## EXAMPLES OF DEFENCE MECHANISMS

Immature defences such as the examples which follow, if over-used, are self-defeating because they are unrewarding, and may be associated with feelings of cynicism and lack of purpose.

a. *Passive aggression* occurs when individuals behave in ways which upset or anger others, without any apparent sign of angry intent. The patient who apparently accepts a treatment plan and then repeatedly fails to comply, or the staff who ignore or treat brusquely an unrewarding or 'difficult' patient may be exhibiting passive aggression.

b. *Rationalisation* is the process of finding the rational explanation (which usually contains a grain of truth) for one's behaviour. Ignoring the intoxicated patient because 'treatment won't help him' or 'we have to treat the more urgent cases first' are common examples. It is important to realise that if such procrastination arises from conscious decision then the staff member is simply being awkward. It is only the immediate, automatic reaction that can be seen as a defence— perhaps against the overt expression of anger or frustration arising out of the feeling of helplessness when faced with such patients.

c.  *Regression* to a less adult way of behaving is common to all illness (staying in bed, being looked after, not going to work) and in severe stress can lead to extremes of muteness, stupor and incontinence.

d.  *Projection* is the unconscious attribution of unrecognised feelings of one's own to others. The addict who is refused a prescription for alleged withdrawal symptoms may say 'You just want to see me suffer—you enjoy it', but this is likely to be an expression of his own anger towards the person seen as withholding necessary treatment.

The following are examples of neurotic defences.

a.  *Dissociation* involves a separation between conscious awareness and part of experience and is the theoretical basis of hysterical conversion (q.v.). It occurs in the face of acute emotional distress and may manifest as amnesia, sudden euphoric or reckless behaviour, fugue states or acute religious fervour.

b.  *Displacement* is the phenomenon whereby the anxiety that is aroused by challenging someone seen as threatening or powerful is avoided by directing anger towards someone weaker. A patient who is irritable and critical towards young student nurses may not be able to confront the consultant or more senior nurses about problems with treatment.

Mature defences such as altruism or humour given as examples below are intrinsically more rewarding than the less mature, and their use may lead to more satisfying conclusions to encounters such as those outlined above.

a.   *Humour* is a widely recognised response to situations in which embarrassment or aggression threaten to disrupt effective cooperation between people.

b.   *Altruism* is when one's own needs are put second to those of others. Delaying lunch to respond rapidly to patients' or staffs' anxiety, even when the situation may not rationally seem to demand an urgent response, can set the scene for better cooperation with later treatment.

c.   *Sublimation* is seen when unrecognised wishes or feelings are diverted into valuable or socially approved activities. The childless person working with children, the person who competes fiercely for promotion and the mild person who 'really likes to get his teeth into' his research may all be using sublimation.

This last example in particular illustrates the danger of over-simplistic interpretations of behaviour. Many factors are involved in determining behaviour, but the styles of response termed defence mechanisms above are widely recognised, not merely in psychological theory but in basic insights found in everyday life, theatre and literature. If health is the use of a wide variety of defences then the habitual overuse of a limited number of defences can become pathological and damaging—for example, use of humour to the extent that it prevents any serious contact with others.

## APPROACHING 'DIFFICULT PATIENTS'

However difficult or intractable a patient's problems might seem to be it is important to remember that an emergency presentation represents an acute failure of normal coping, and this failure needs to be understood and appropriate responses formulated. A clear, structured approach provides the best way to avoid the dangers outlined above.

## 1. SUPPORT AND UNDERSTANDING

The approach to the patient should always represent an attempt to understand him as an individual with specific problems. Powerful feelings that interfere with this, such as anger, embarrassment or misery should be dealt with by reflecting them back to the patient in an attempt to understand them further ('I can see you're angry, could you tell my why'). Rather than feeling 'overdoses just waste my time' both patient and doctor will get more satisfaction from 'If I can understand what happened I might be able to help'.

## 2. STRUCTURE AND LIMIT SETTING

a. The nature and purpose of the interview, the time available and the conditions under which the interviewer feels able to help with the patient's problems should be clearly stated ('I can't really offer much while you're shouting at me, why don't you take a minute or two to calm down and I'll come back and talk then').

b. If the conditions are clearly unacceptable to the patient they should, within limits, be negotiable, but should be kept to once agreed, and if necessary restated at intervals.

c. If patients do not cooperate with the wishes of the interviewer he/she should attempt to understand why ('It's obvious you don't feel able to sit still and talk— perhaps if I left the door open and you can pace up and down you'd be able to tell me a little more about what's going on?').

d. All interviews should begin with open-ended questions about the immediate difficulties, but control can be kept by increasingly closed or directive questions as the problem becomes clearer ('I'll come back to whether drugs are the right treatment later, but before that could you tell me how you've been sleeping?').

e. Patients who present with inconsistent or unbelievable stories, or bizarre ideas are best met with puzzled concern ('I'm afraid I don't understand—you say the anxiety's only been bad for a few days, but you've been taking tablets for it for two years. Why's that?') or agreement to differ ('I understand why you're frightened if you feel that aliens are trying to kill you, but I guess you know that I don't really share those ideas'). The extremes of open confrontation or dishonest acceptance ('humouring') are best avoided.

## 3. AVOIDING CONFLICT

Sometimes inteviewer and patient seem to be irreconcilably at odds, for example the patient insists on being given drugs, or being admitted, or continues to behave in an aggressive or uncooperative fashion. At such times getting into arguments is pointless. Alternatives include:

a. Redirecting the interview onto more fruitful lines ('You keep mentioning how fed up your husband's getting—is this making you more upset?').

b. Enlisting the patient's cooperation in solving the problem ('We seem to be at odds over this—I don't think medication is going to help you solve your problems, but you feel you can't do without it. Let's try and find something that we'll both think is helpful').

c. Stopping the interview for a short time. This time can be used by both interviewer and patient to calm down and defuse unhelpful emotions. It may also give the interviewer time to discuss the case with other staff who can provide a more objective framework for understanding and coping with the patient.

## 4. OTHER STAFF AND INFORMANTS

Some patients arouse conflicting feelings in staff, or play off one staff member against another. Good communication between staff is essential and management plans should be agreed with clear guidelines about who is responsible for which aspects of management.

Other sources of information (old notes, other staff, relatives, previous and present doctors involved) may be able to provide useful information, experience and suggestions that can resolve problems that otherwise seem insoluble.

Any treatment plan involving other agencies must be agreed by all concerned before it is offered to the patient.

# Part B
# Syndromes presenting as emergencies

# 4. Acute psychoses

The term acute psychosis refers to the relatively sudden onset of a disturbance in the patient's grasp of reality. The patient makes false judgements about the nature of his perceptions or thoughts even in the face of evidence to the contrary. Acute psychosis is not a diagnosis but the description of a clinical syndrome found in a variety of disorders (*see Table* 4.1).

The acute psychotic syndrome develops rapidly over days or weeks. There will be reports of a deteriorating level of occupational and social function and possibly personal hygiene. The symptoms of acute psychosis include seriously disorganised behaviour, bizarre beliefs, hallucinations and incoherent speech (*see Table* 4.2).

As well as agitation and hyperactivity there may be poor self-control and loss of judgement. These impairments may lead to violence, accidental or deliberate self-harm or serious social problems (arrest, loss of job, damage to close relationships), and so acute psychoses should be viewed as medical emergencies and responded to appropriately.


## DIAGNOSIS

It is usually fairly easy to recognise an acute psychosis. The patient may be so 'mad' and disorganised that the condition is immediately apparent. The history may be nonsensical or hard to follow. The patient may admit to hallucinations or appear to be hearing or seeing things the interviewer cannot perceive.

The differential diagnosis of specific causes of the acute psychosis may be more difficult. The history may be impossible to take from the patient so other informants should be consulted.

As an absolute minimum the history should include:

*Table* 4.1. ILLNESSES WHICH MAY PRESENT AS AN ACUTE
PSYCHOSIS

Affective disorders—mania or agitated depression
Acute onset of schizophrenia
Relapse of chronic schizophrenia
Hallucinogen and amphetamine abuse
Withdrawal from alcohol or barbiturates
Acute confusional states (delirium)

*Table* 4.2. THE SYMPTOMS OF ACUTE PSYCHOSIS

| Disorder | Symptoms and signs |
| --- | --- |
| Thought | Delusions; ideas of reference; incoherence; loose associations |
| Speech | Conveys little information; circumstantial; rambling; incoherent |
| Perception | Hallucinations; illusions; depersonalisation; derealisation |
| Mood | Labile; inappropriate; extremes of euphoria, depression or anger |
| Behaviour | Disorganisation; hyperactivity; psychomotor agitation or retardation; impulsivity. |

1. The course of the current illness—symptoms, onset and duration, sleep and appetite disturbance.
2. Past history—age of onset, duration of illness episodes, level of functioning before onset and in remission, past response to treatment.
3. Medical history—especially of cerebrovascular disease, endocrine disorders, hepatic or renal disease and fits.
4. Medication—currrent and past.
5. Drug and alcohol use—current and past.
6. Family history—mental illness, alcoholism or neurological disease.

## EMERGENCY TREATMENT

Acutely psychotic patients can be difficult to treat in an emergency setting as they are often over-aroused and disruptive, may be irritable and unpredictable and not responsive to reason or persuasion. The fear that this arouses in staff can lead to these patients being left alone, or confronted, perhaps by police or security guards. Such angry or fearful responses tend to make the patient more anxious and disruptive and a vicious cycle begins.

There is a temptation to label disturbed patients as 'psychiatric' (especially if there has been a 'precipitating' cause such as a recent stressful event), sedate them immediately and dispose of them rapidly without proper consideration of the aetiology of the psychosis. Immediate sedation can lead to dangerous misjudgements such as missing medical or neurological illnesses. All patients should have a full physical examination performed before a final decision about diagnosis is made.

The first responsibility of whoever is in charge is to ensure the safety of both patient and staff (*see* Chapter 10). Ensuring the safety of the patient includes not leaving until a full assessment has been made.

### 1. APPROACH TO THE PATIENT

The immediate aim of emergency treatment must be the reduction of symptoms such as agitation, anxiety, aggression and poor impulse control. This can often be achieved by approaching the patient and his problems in a calm and systematic way.

Approaches to mute or unresponsive patients are discussed in another chapter (*see* Chapter 9), but in general a calm and patient approach with empathic interventions ('I can see it's hard to talk' or 'You look very frightened when I talk to you, I wonder what that's about?') will often draw withdrawn patients out.

Paranoid patients may also refuse to talk, or be very suspicious or hostile. Consistency, respect and calm should be the hallmarks of the interviewer's approach. The patients should be allowed to express some of their anger or suspiciousness, but within limits ('I can see that's made you very angry, but now there are a few things I'd like to discuss with you'). Head on confrontation, responding to the patient's anger and getting into fruitless arguments (especially about issues of blame, or the precise details of events) are only too easy with such patients, but must be avoided.

## 2. USE OF MEDICATION

Many patients will calm down with the approach described above, and in these cases pharmacological management should be avoided. Agitated or severely disturbed patients will require admission to a psychiatric ward and there is little purpose in giving large doses of neuroleptics before admission. An outline of procedures for emergency tranquillisation in disturbed or aggressive patients is given in Chapter 18.

## THE FUNCTIONAL PSYCHOSES

Functional (non-organic) psychoses are distinguished from those in which there is a known or presumed organic aetiology (organic psychoses—q.v.). Functional psychoses include schizophrenic disorders, affective disorders and paranoid psychoses. In an emergency situation it is rarely necessary to do more than establish that a psychosis is functional rather than organic. It may be helpful to be aware of the characteristics of the main functional psychoses, which are outlined briefly below, with indications of specific ways in which they may present.

## 1. SCHIZOPHRENIA

Schizophrenia may present as an acute first episode of illness, or as part of a severe disorder of long duration. Relapses are commonly due to non-compliance with medication or social or family stress. Psychotic symptoms occur in clear consciousness, a feature distinguishing schizophrenia from acute confusional states (q.v.).

a. There may be *abnormal motor activity*, with retardation or agitation.
b. *Rapport* is difficult to establish.
c. *Speech* may be circumstantial, contain odd or unusual words and phrases or be almost incomprehensible.
d. *Mood* is often depressed or anxious, but may be blunted, flat or inappropriate.
e. *Thought* content may include delusions or ideas of reference not consistent with the prevailing mood. There may be disorders of the possession of thought such as thought broadcasting (the belief that others are sharing or listening to the patient's thoughts), thought insertion (the experience of alien thoughts being put into one's mind) and thought withdrawal (the experience of thoughts being removed from one's mind, often attributed to an outside agency).
f. *Perceptual disturbances* most commonly take the form of auditory hallucinations. If these take the form of commands there is the danger that they might be acted on, and they should be taken at face value.

## 2. MANIA

a. *Mood* may be euphoric, or infectiously cheerful, but more often than not the patient is irritable, or his mood is labile and unpredictable.
b. *Behaviour, talk* and *thought* are characteristically speeded up.
c. The patient does not sleep, is over-active and energetic. Activity is usually disorganised, for example patients may not eat because they are too disorganised to stay long enough at the table.

d. Patients may *act impulsively*, with poor judgement, for example writing large cheques their bank account will not cover for goods they do not need. They may be disinhibited (including sexual disinhibition) with poor social judgement.

e. *Thinking* includes grandiose ideas or delusions; there may be pressure of talk and flight of ideas. Disturbances of perception are not common.

f. The clinical picture may be confused by drugs or alcohol that the patient has been using to excess in an attempt to control his mood swings.

Manic patients characteristically feel well and have little or no insight. They will probably have been brought in unwillingly, and may be on bad terms with whoever brought them. It is best to see the patient without the person accompanying them at first, and any discussion with another informant should be done with the patient present if possible. It is possible to acknowledge the patient's high spirits without getting caught up in the mood and responding to the gaiety and joking. Manic patients love an audience, but will respond better to a professional who has retained his professional stance.

## 3. DEPRESSIVE PSYCHOSIS

Depressive psychosis is the affective counterpart of mania, and is the extreme pole of the spectrum of severity of depressive illness. Depression rarely presents with over-arousal and over-activity, but some patients may present with agitation or paranoid features.

a. *Mood* will be low.

b. *'Biological' symptoms* (poor appetite, weight loss, sleep disturbance, lowered libido, tiredness and decreased energy, poor concentration) will be present.

c. *Self-denigration*, guilt, feelings of personal worthlessness and suicidal ideation are common.

  d. *Mood congruent delusions* may be present, such as
     beliefs of deserved persecution, or of guilt and impend-
     ing punishment. There may be delusions of disease,
     such as the belief that parts of the body have rotted
     away.
  e. *Hallucinations* are typically persecutory or insulting
     ('You're no good' or 'It's all your fault') and may give
     the patient instructions to kill themselves. These may
     be acted on and should be taken very seriously.

Depressed patients may have slowed thoughts and poor
concentration, making the interview difficult. The interviewer should be patient, and his questions straightforward,
simple and related to symptoms ('How is your appetite?').
The interviewer should be active, but responsive to the
patient's mood ('You seem to be very low at present. Have
you found yourself thinking that life isn't worth living?'). In
extreme cases of depressive stupor, the patient may be
completely mute and unresponsive.

Depressed patients are at high risk of suicide; assessment
and treatment must take this into account (*see* Chapter 16).
Severely depressed patients require hospitalisation so there is
no need to prescribe medication as an emergency treatment.
Antidepressant drugs can exacerbate psychotic symptoms
and should only be given after admission when the patient's
state can be properly monitored.


## 4. PARANOID STATES

Paranoid disorders are characterised by persistent delusions
occuring in clear consciousness. Delusions are usually
persecutory (feeling spied upon, threatened or plotted
against) but may involve other beliefs (for example, delusions
of jealousy). These delusions severely disrupt social
and family functioning, but the patient's intellect is not
affected and (surprisingly) he may continue with his normal
occupation.

Paranoid patients rarely have insight into their illness and so do not come seeking treatment. They may be brought unwillingly by relatives, or present with a story of injustice or persecution for the interviewer to deal with, while denying that they wish treatment.

## 5. MORBID JEALOUSY

A paranoid illness of particular importance, although rare, is morbid jealousy (q.v.), where the patient (usually male) believes his sexual partner is being unfaithful and may go to extreme lengths to check on this belief or prevent the supposed infidelity. The importance of this condition lies in the fact that it can lead to homicide of the partner or (less commonly) her supposed lover.

Paranoid patients are often hostile and suspicious, and may be litiginous. Dealing with paranoid patients can be particulary difficult and care must be taken not to get embroiled in angry disputation.

## 6. FEIGNED PSYCHOSIS

Very rarely patients present with a feigned psychotic illness. This presentation may be seen in patients brought in by police after arrest and is an attempt to avoid jail and prosecution. It may also be a psychological variant of Munchausen's syndrome (q.v.). However, there is evidence that the majority of patients thought to be feigning psychosis eventually go on to a diagnosis of chronic psychotic illness.

In feigned psychosis symptoms do not fit the pattern of established psychiatric diagnoses. Characteristically responses to cognitive function testing are wrong in a pattern indicating the patient is aware of the correct response and is giving 'approximate' answers rather than inappropriate or meaningless ones—for example saying the reigning monarch is 'King Philip' or getting simple arithmetical problems slightly wrong in a systematic way. Symptoms may vary with the situation, getting worse when the patient knows he is being observed.

The distinction between feigned and actual psychosis can be difficult to make and if there is any doubt psychiatric admission for assessment should be arranged. Confronting the patient with the belief he is feigning illness is of no value in management.

## ADMISSION TO HOSPITAL

Recognising acute psychosis is usually not a major problem, but deciding on and organising treatment can be difficult and is invariably time-consuming. Any further care, but especially involuntary hospitalisation, will require the help and support of relatives and friends if available, so it is worth spending time with them summarising and explaining the problem and the treatment offered.

Acutely psychotic patients will usually require admission to a psychiatric unit. Admission is definitely indicated:

1. In a first psychotic illness.
2. If the patient is endangering himself (suicidal or neglectful of his safety in dangerous situations for instance) or presents a danger to others (for example, threatening revenge on persecutors).
3. If an organic aetiology is suspected.
4. If there is inadequate or absent family and social support.
5. If there is a history of poor compliance with treatment during previous illness episodes.
6. If the patient's judgement or insight are so poor as to threaten the efficacy of treatment.

Reasons for hospitalisation should be expressed in terms of illness and treatment ('Your mood is very high at present and that's making it difficult for you to control your actions') rather than it being seen as a punishment for unacceptable behaviour ('You have to go into hospital to stop you hitting your mother again'). In the main patients will accept admission willingly, but there are some occasions that a patient may have to be admitted to or detained in hospital against his will under the mental health legislation (*see* Chapter 20).

## OUT-PATIENT CARE

If none of the indications for admission are met then it may be possible to treat the patient as an out-patient. There should be positive reasons for this decision, such as good family support or a history of previously successful out-patient management. Information about past responses to medication and treatment of relapse should be obtained where possible from case notes, doctors who know the patient or involved family and friends. Follow-up must be adequately planned.

*Before* the patient leaves, whoever is responsible for organising follow-up should ensure that:

1. All arrangements that have been made have been discussed in detail with the patient and other responsible persons.
2. The follow-up arrangements include:
    a. prescription of appropriate medication;
    b. ensuring the patient is referred to a psychiatrist within 48 hours;
    c. ensuring that both the patient and a responsible other person know how to contact emergency services should they require to do so.
3. Other individuals or agencies involved in the plan have been contacted and have agreed to their role.

(Modified from Hanke, 1984.)

Any medication prescribed should be sufficient to alleviate distressing symptoms until psychiatric out-patient care can be obtained. Haloperidol is less sedating and has fewer acute side effects than other neuroleptics. An appropriate dose would be 5–10 mg four times daily. The patient may well know which drug suits him best, and in what doses. It is not advisable to give antiparkinsonian medication prophylactically, but the patient should be warned about possible side effects and instructed to return if extrapyramidal effects prove troublesome. Acute dystonias can be treated with procyclidine 10 mg parenterally or orally.

# 5. Psychiatric presentations of organic brain disease

A group of disorders characterised by a global decrease in intellectual functioning sufficient to interfere with performance of normal social or occupational roles are referred to as the organic brain syndromes (OBS). These include delirium and dementia, amnestic syndromes, intoxicated states and toxic psychoses due to drug use or withdrawal. Patients present with psychiatric or behavioural abnormalities which are associated with transient or permanent cerebral dysfunction.

Psychiatric symptoms in organic brain syndromes may be due to actual brain damage or to the patient's reaction to his own awareness of failing cognitive function.

Patients with organic brain syndromes are often referred because of agitated and bizarre behaviour, possibly with unusual perceptual experiences or beliefs. Assessment may be less thorough when the reasons for mental and behavioural changes are assumed, for example, the presumptive diagnosis of intoxication in someone who smells of alcohol. Physical complaints may be ignored or given little importance. Premature psychiatric referral is often made because these patients can be frustrating or annoying to deal with, especially those who may be seen as 'to blame' for their condition (e.g. alcoholics and drug addicts). However, failure to recognise organic causes for symptoms does the patient a grave disservice, and can be life-threatening.

Criteria strongly suggesting the presence of organic disease are:

a. disorientation;
b. clouded consciousness;
c. age over 40 with no past psychiatric history;
d. visual hallucinations or illusions;
e. abnormal vital signs.

Minimal physical examination must include checking vital signs, looking for signs of head injury (bruising; blood in ears; csf rhinorrhoea) and looking for unequal or dilated pupils. Nystagmus, ophthalmoplegia and ataxia can also be observed during the interview. If the patient will cooperate—and with a calm, systematic approach most will—then evidence of abnormalities in the fundi, neck rigidity, and systemic disorders (GI; pulmonary; renal; hepatic) must be sought.

Essential urgent special investigations include: FBC and differential; ESR; urinalysis; urea and electrolytes; blood sugar; chest X-ray; serum calcium; ECG.

Distinguishing between acute and chronic brain syndromes is not always easy, and in this text we prefer to distinguish delirious from dementing states, while warning that these are not entirely synonymous with acute and chronic syndromes. It should be remembered that these terms describe clinical syndromes, *not* diagnoses, and diagnosis in aetiological terms must be avidly pursued.

## DELIRIUM (SYNONYMS: ACUTE CONFUSIONAL STATE; ACUTE OBS)

Delirium refers to a global impairment of cerebral function, generally characterised by rapid onset (6 hr-4 days), fluctuating course and relatively brief duration. In the majority of cases the symptoms are completely reversible. Onset can be at any age, and may be sudden or following a prodromal stage lasting hours or days. During the prodromal stage the patient may develop restlessness, insomnia, nightmares, have trouble

*Table* 5.1: CAUSES OF ACUTE CONFUSIONAL STATES (DELIRIUM)

| Cause | Examples |
|---|---|
| Infections | Meningitis; encephalitis; brain abscess; pneumonia; neurosyphilis; any systemic infection in elderly |
| Drug withdrawal | Alchohol; sedative-hypnotics |
| Drug toxicity | Digitalis; methyldopa; anticholinergics; antiparkinsonian agents; antidepressants sedatives; antihistamines; alcohol; anticonvulsants; hallucinogens; amphetamine; cimetidine; narcotic analgesics; steroids |
| Hypoxia | Pneumonia; COAD; pulmonary embolus; 'silent' MI |
| Endocrine | Hypoglycaemia; ketoacidosis; hyperthyroidism; hyperparathyroidism; adrenal insufficiency |
| Metabolic | Hepatic encephalopathy; uraemia; thiamine deficiency; B12 and folate 'deficiency; electrolyte disturbances; porphyria |
| Neoplastic | Brain tumour; cerebral metastases |
| Intracranial | Haemorrhage (subdural in elderly, alcoholics); head injury; cerebrovascular lesions; cerebral vasculitis (SLE, PAN, temporal arteritis) |
| Degenerative | Alzheimer's and other dementias; multiple sclerosis |

thinking clearly and be hypersensitive to environmental stimuli. Some causes of delirium are given in *Table* 5.1.

*Physical examination* may be normal except for signs of autonomic overactivity (blood pressure, heart rate, respiratory rate, and temperature are all increased) and sometimes tremor.

## MENTAL STATE

Mental state examination is marked by lability and inconsistency of mood, activity and perception. Level of consciousness is reduced, there is disorientation and short-term memory is severely impaired.

a. *Clouding of consciousness* is prominent. Clouding refers to an impaired clarity in the patient's awareness of the environment. This can vary (between patients or in the same patient) from minimal impairment through somnolence to coma. The patient shows reduced ability to shift, focus or sustain attention. It is important to distinguish clouding of consciousness from lack of cooperation.

b. *Behaviour.* There is a change in psychomotor activity which may range from sluggish or stuporose to restless and agitated. The sleep cycle is disturbed or reversed. There may be insomnia, nightmares, daytime drowsiness and nocturnal hyperalertness.

c. *Impulse control and judgement* are usually severely impaired. Patients may be combative, paranoid and obstinate.

d. *Speech* can be rambling, fragmented, perseverative or incoherent. Patients may move from topic to topic in a disjointed way.

e. *Mood* is often labile (e.g. moving from fear to tearfulness to calm in a few minutes). Patients can show a range of emotions including fear, anxiety, irritability, apathy, depression or euphoria.

f. *Perception.* There may be perceptual disturbances; both sensation and recognition can be affected. Sensory misperceptions are common, for example failing to recognise familiar people or claiming recognition of unfamiliar staff as close relatives. There may be illusions or fragmentary hallucinations. These are typically visual and colourful; tactile hallucinations should also suggest organic disease. Olfactory hallucinations may be associated with temporal lobe fits.

g. *Thought* patterns are disorganised and incoherent. There may be delusions which are typically shallow, rapidly changing and lacking detail.

h. *Intellectual functions.* Patients are severely disorientated in time and often in place and person; short-term memory is usually severely impaired.

All the above symptoms can fluctuate, usually becoming worse at night. Patients may well be lucid in the morning, and this can be a trap for the unwary interviewer who sees the patient at this time and pays too little attention to the history or other informants.

Delirious states usually last about one week, but in elderly patients may take many weeks to clear. Full recovery is the most common outcome but some progress to chronic organic brain syndromes (e.g. Korsakov's psychosis following Wernicke's encephalopathy) and some patients die, particularly if the organic aetiology is unrecognised.

Several conditions have been identified as potentially life threatening or having very severe consequences, causing irreversible brain damage. The following conditions require emergency treatment if they are suspected (NB: the typical features described may not be pronounced and can easily be overlooked):

1. Meningitis and encephalitis—headache, fever, neck rigidity, leucocytosis.
2. Hypoglycaemia—pallor, sweating, rapid pulse.
3. Diabetic ketoacidosis or hyperosmolality—flushing, hyperventilation.
4. Hypoxia and anoxia—history of acute pulmonary or cardiac disease. Chronic disease with superimposed mild pneumonia or CCF.
5. Hyperthermia—raised temperature.
6. Wernicke's encephalopathy—ataxia, ophthalmoplegia and memory loss.
7. Hypertensive encephalopathy—severe headache followed by confusion. High blood pressure.
8. Intracranial haemorrhage—focal neurological signs.

## DEMENTIA (SYNONYM: CHRONIC OBS)

Dementia refers to a clinical syndrome characterised by global intellectual impairment leading to loss of social and occupational functioning in a setting of *clear consciousness*. It may not be immediately apparent as patients often retain social and conversational skills but these are soon discovered to be superficial and cover impairments in memory, abstract thinking, social judgement, higher cortical functions and personality.

For definite diagnosis there should be evidence of an organic factor, but this can be assumed if the patient satisfies the diagnosis clinically and 'reversible' aetiologies (*see Table 5.2*) have been excluded.

*Table* 5.2: CAUSES OF DEMENTIA

| Cause | Examples |
|---|---|
| *Reversible* | |
| Drugs | Alcohol; barbiturates |
| Depression | |
| Trauma | Subdural haematoma; normal pressure hydro-cephalus |
| Infection | Syphilis; encephalitis |
| Vitamin deficiencies | Thiamine; niacin; B12; folic acid |
| Endocrine | Thyroid; parathyroid; hypoglycaemia |
| Vascular | Carotid occlusion; cranial arteritis |
| Metabolic disorders | Wilson's disease; calcium or electrolyte disturbance; cardiac failure; renal failure; hepatic insufficiency |
| Tumour | |
| *Irreversible (only if others excluded)* | |
| Degenerative | Senile dementia; Alzheimer's disease; Pick's disease; Huntington's chorea; multiple sclerosis |
| Trauma | Repeated head injury (e.g. boxers) |
| Vascular | Multi infarct dementia |

Demented patients can be extremely trying for staff in emergency settings. This is because the presentation is frequently due to social or other factors only secondarily related to the dementia, and usually not seen by the staff as medical emergencies. There is a tendency to try to solve the problem by referral to another agency, perhaps a psychiatrist, and this can in turn lead to friction and argument.

Another problem faced by staff dealing with demented patients is the common belief that all conditions are chronic, progressive and irreversible. This produces an attitude of therapeutic nihilism, and ignores the 30–40% of cases in whom intervention can provide some help.

*Case example:* An elderly woman was brought to the casualty department by distraught relatives, who complained that she had become increasingly confused, irritable and suspicious and that they could no longer cope with her. On examination she had profound short-term memory loss, and was agitated and irritable. Orientation was not assessed. The duty psychiatrist was contacted and asked to admit the patient, but he discovered recent case notes indicating that the patient had been seen two days previously by a consultant psychogeriatrician, who found no evidence of an acute disturbance. The duty psychiatrist suggested that the patient be sent home, and implied that the family were not accepting their responsibility for caring for the patient. Two days later the patient was seen by the psychogeriatrician who admitted her as an emergecny with severe pneumonia.

The patient's *appearance* and *behaviour* may show signs of impaired social judgement, as exhibited by neglect of dress or appearance, bad language, inappropriate or impulsive behaviour.

The patient's *mood* may be labile, and a common presentation in the early stages of dementia is with intractable depression, anxiety or nervousness. There may be withdrawal and irritability. The patient may produce multiple somatic complaints, and there may be a history of extensive negative physical investigation.

The most prominent loss is usually in *memory*. In mild cases patients tend to forget the events of the day, or show hesitancy in answering questions about their activities. As the syndrome becomes more severe, patients begin regularly to forget the names of things or people, and become unable to learn new information. They increasingly reminisce about the past, but eventually memory for past events is impaired, and the patient may forget to complete tasks they are engaged in, for example regularly leaving kettles or pans to boil dry. Tests of intellectual function show failure of short-term memory.

Mental state examination will also reveal evidence of impaired abstract thinking.

Relatives will probably describe a change in the patient's *personality*. Personality traits may be exaggerated (e.g. suspiciousness becoming paranoia) or reversed (e.g. orderliness giving way to disorder and self-neglect). The patient may exhibit reduced awareness of the needs or feelings of others, manners may deteriorate and behaviour might be socially inappropriate (for example, shoplifting, indecency). There is loss of interest in the surroundings with repetitiveness in conversation and thought; patients may adopt a rigid schedule and become very agitated if their routine is disturbed. Patients frequently wander or get lost. There is a risk of accidental self-harm.

Incontinence, aphasia, apraxia, agnosia or other frank *neurological signs* develop in the latter stages of the illness.

Demented patients are more vulnerable to infections, and to developing delirious states. Death is usually secondary to medical complications. Many dementias are potentially reversible and treatable (*see Table* 5.2).

Dementia needs to be differentiated from delirium (both states can co-exist) and so-called 'pseudodementia'.

The term *pseudodementia* is controversial and poorly defined, but there is no doubt that in some patients presenting with memory impairment, poor concentration and poor performance on cognitive tests these can be symptoms of depressive illness which may go unrecognised. Diagnostic features of this condition are primary disturbance of mood (depressed or irritable), biological symptoms of depression (q.v.), definite time of onset, and relatively rapid progression of symptoms. There is often variable performance on cognitive testing and patients show marked distress over impairments thus detected. The symptoms do not fluctuate or get worse at night.

If there is any doubt it is best to treat patients for depression while completing the appropriate investigations for dementia.


## AMNESTIC SYNDROMES

These are profound impairments in the ability to form new memories which occur in *clear consciousness*. There is bilateral damage to diencephalic and medial temporal structures such as the hippocampus and mamillary bodies. Common causes of amnestic syndromes are head injury, infections, hypoxia, infarction, and Korsakov's psychosis (q.v.).


## ACUTE INTOXICATION

Acute intoxication with drugs or alcohol is a common condition, so common it tends not to be thought of as an organic brain syndrome. These conditions are dealt with elsewhere (q.v.) and mentioned here for completeness.


## DIAGNOSIS

Obtaining a detailed history and mental state can be difficult if the patient is confused, uncooperative or belligerent. The structure of the interview and its situation can make all the difference between obtaining an adequate history and one that is diagnostically useless.

The situation and the nature and purpose of the interview should be explained in simple language. The interview itself needs structuring. If open ended questions elicit little information or provoke anxiety or confusion they should rapidly be replaced by questions directing the patient to specific topics.

Patients may try to avoid cognitive testing by, for example, jokes and evasiveness. Each step in the assessment of cognitive function should be explained to the patient and then performed with polite insistence unless the patient becomes too distressed ('catastrophe reaction').

The most important sign in delirium is disorientation. Loss of orientation for time, day, month, year, place and person occur in that order as the severity of the disturbance increases.

Any relatives or others present will have to be involved early in the assessment. They should be asked about previous medical and psychiatric illnesses, current medication or drug abuse, the onset and course of the symptoms, what changes they have observed in the patient and any previous similar episodes. A history of drowsiness, ataxia, dysarthria or incontinence, or fluctuations in the severity of the symptoms should be considered strong indicators of an organic aetiology.

## TREATMENT

### 1. GENERAL PROBLEMS

Effective treatment of patients with organic syndromes can be hampered by conflicts arising between professionals about who should provide the most appropriate treatment. Psychiatric staff are skilled in the management of agitation and disturbed behaviour, but frequently feel that other special- ised medical input is required for medical conditions, especially if these are serious or life-threatening. Too commonly each side in such disputes imagines that skills they take for granted are easy for the other, failing to recognise their own anxieties. Such conflicts should be avoided and it must be recognised that medical and psychiatric teams (and possibly others such as neurosurgeons) have joint responsibility.

## 2. ENVIRONMENT

The patient should be offered quiet and privacy in a well-lit room, avoiding over-stimulation by keeping activity to a minimum. A family member or someone the patient knows should remain present. The patient should be addressed politely by his name and title, and any staff should introduce themselves. The number of strange people the patient meets should be restricted. One interviewer and one nurse should be the maximum—avoid crowds of medical students, or rapid changes of nurse. Any procedures should be explained and the patient should be regularly reorientated by reminding him of where he is, the name and function of staff, and so forth.

## 3. MEDICATION

Drug treatment should be avoided in the emergency setting wherever possible. The clinical picture may well be confused by tranquillisers, and cognitive function made worse. Agitation, irritability and impulsivity are the symptoms most likely to provoke a response using drugs, but these symptoms are often improved by the non-specific treatments outlined above. If these fail then sedation may need to be used cautiously.

Neuroleptics are generally safe, and can be used in low doses for rapid control of agitation and anxiety without worsening delirium, but they can cause severe hypotension or induce epileptic fits. Benzodiazepines have minimal cardiovascular effects, but may increase confusion or disinhibited behaviour. Benzodiazepines are specifically contraindicated in pulmonary disease, severe renal disease and porphyria. Sedation may mask important symptoms and should be avoided if there is any evidence of reduced level of consciousness.

## 4. FURTHER MANAGEMENT

All delirious patients should be admitted to hospital for investigation and treatment. No patient should be discharged while still confused, or if a definite diagnosis has not been made.

Dementia should never be diagnosed for the first time in an emergency setting, most especially in the presenium. Most cases will need to be admitted for full assessment. However, most demented patients present as emergencies with acute social difficulties or with minor changes that do not require hospitalisation but have caused the home situation to become intolerable. These situations can often be dealt with without admitting the patient. Such patients need the support of their families or other agencies, and effective intervention in the emergency setting can often help to re-establish such support. Before the patient leaves the following must be arranged and discussed with both the patient and his relatives:

a. *Medication:* Symptomatic treatment can be given for anxiety, agitation, or depression. Elderly demented patients are especially sensitive to side-effects, so doses must be kept small, and if circumstances permit a test dose can be offered. Moderate anxiety is probably best treated with benzodiazepines, while more severe agitation or frank paranoia will require a neuroleptic. A neuroleptic offered for a few nights can re-establish a normal sleep pattern. A family member must agree to be in charge of dispensing medication. Both the patient and his relatives should be informed of possible side-effects, and be aware how to obtain urgent advice should there be problems.

b. *Support:* Family members will be the most usual source of support, but neighbours, voluntary agencies, etc., may take the burden, or provide relief for over-burdened families.

c. *Follow-up:* If necessary arrangements must be made for full investigation of the causes of dementia. Referral to a psychogeriatrician may be helpful if there are severe or enduring psychiatric symptoms. Medical social workers are an invaluable source of information about, for example, luncheon clubs, day centres, meals on wheels, nursing homes and other support agencies. The patient may need referral for day care.

# 6.   Disorders related to anxiety

Intolerable anxiety is the driving force behind all emergency presentations. Whatever has occurred, the patient or a significant other person feels that the problem is beyond their capacity to cope and that delay obtaining help would be intolerable. It is essential that anyone who routinely has to deal with emergency situations is familiar with the effects of anxiety both on the patient and on others, and with techniques for dealing with it.

Anxiety is a powerful and extremely distressing emotion. Those in the grip of severe anxiety feel panic, apprehension and desperation, without any clear understanding of why they feel this way. These feelings are accompanied by an overwhelming wish to do something about them. People in the grip of anxiety cannot sleep, find their thoughts racing, cannot concentrate, are constantly alert for danger and may fear for their sanity. They are restless and overactive; they pace up and down, or find jobs to do such as incessant cleaning and tidying. They cannot tolerate being alone, and may demand the company of friends or relatives. They actively seek out help, usually asking impatiently for immediate relief from their distress.

Anxiety is contagious, and the patient's behaviour and demands can become irritating or frustrating. Staff will be affected by these feelings as well and it is essential that they remain composed and in command.

## PRESENTATION

General symptoms of anxiety (*see Table* 6.1) include disturbances of mood and a variety of physical symptoms and signs, many of which are consequences of autonomic arousal.

*Table* 6.1. SYMPTOMS AND SIGNS OF ANXIETY

| | |
|---|---|
| Mood | Apprehension; dread; fear; impatience; irritability; panic; jitteriness |
| Skin | Sweating; pallor |
| Gastrointestinal | Dry mouth; lump in the throat; abdominal cramps; nausea; anorexia; diarrhoea |
| Motor system | Muscle tension; restlessness; tremulousness; pacing |
| Cardiovascular | Palpitations; tachycardia; syncope; chest pain |
| Respiratory | Tightness in chest; shortness of breath |
| Neurological | Dizziness; paraesthesia; headache; tension; vertigo; weakness |
| Psychological | Obsessions; compulsions; depersonalisation; derealisation; phobias; ruminations |

Anxiety or panic states are common, and may present in a variety of ways. A common presentation is with somatic symptoms, for example chest pain or dyspnoea. Patients may be brought by others who mistake a panic attack for a heart attack. Severe anxiety may bring a patient to believe they are seriously ill or dying, and these beliefs may be based on physiological symptoms of anxiety, for example chest pain or difficulty drawing breath. Symptoms of hyperventilation such as dizziness, dyspnoea and paraesthesia are common reasons for presentation. Often negative physical investigations lead to the patient being dismissed with the idea there is 'nothing really wrong'. Distressing or incapacitating symptoms are dismissed as hysterical. This is a grave failure to understand the degree of distress and to institute appropriate treatment measures.

The anxiety itself can become incapacitating, especially if social support is reduced, for example a close relative being admitted to hospital, and the patient may present as being unable to cope, or with suicidal ideation.

Finally the patient may be brought by others who find the patient's symptoms or demanding behaviour intolerable.

## CAUSES OF ANXIETY

Anxiety is a common state which can be a normal response to threatening external events. Anxiety is reasonable in response to the illness of a family member, or when faced with imminent examinations, and panic may be experienced in situations of grave danger over which there is no control, for example in a car skidding at speed on ice.

External threats which commonly provoke anxiety which the patient experiences as having no obvious cause are losses, including those by death or separation, and conflicts with others, often in situations of physical closeness, for example in families.

*Case example:* The husband of a woman admitted to an orthopaedic ward with a compound fracture of the leg pestered staff to discharge his wife prematurely and demanded that her treatment be speeded up. Shortly afterwards he presented at the casualty department with extreme anxiety, complaining he was 'unable to cope', despite the fact that his children were being cared for by a neighbour.

Symptoms of anxiety can be a consequence of physical illnesss or drug use. There are many medical illnesses that can present with physiological symptoms of anxiety, often associated with fear and nervousness (*see Table* 6.2) and it is important that these be excluded in the differential diagnosis of anxiety states. It is not unknown for patients with a pulmonary embolus or myocardial infarction to be treated for anxiety and the primary diagnosis missed.

Finally, anxiety is associated with many psychiatric disorders, for example depression, mania, acute psychoses. In addition the effects of psychotropic medication need to be considered. Akathisia may be produced by neuroleptic medication, and antidepressants may cause tachycardias and arousal. Both these side-effects can be mistaken for anxiety states.

*Table* 6.2. PHYSIOLOGICAL CAUSES OF ANXIETY

| | |
|---|---|
| Cardiovascular | Angina pectoris |
| | Myocardial infarction |
| | Mitral valve prolapse |
| | Paroxysmal supraventricular tachycardia |
| Respiratory | Acute respiratory distress |
| | Pulmonary embolism |
| | Asthma |
| Endocrine | Hypoglcyaemia |
| | Thyrotoxicosis |
| | Phaeochromocytoma |
| Neurological | Delirium |
| | Epilepsy (esp. psychomotor) |
| | Stroke |
| Psychophysiological | Pain or serious threat |
| Medication | L-dopa |
| | Steriods |
| | Thyroxine |
| | Bronchodilators |

## SPECIFIC STATES ASSOCIATED WITH ANXIETY

1. *Panic attacks* are discrete episodes of intense, sometimes disabling, anxiety or terror, with associated physical symptoms (*see Table* 6.1). They display rapid onset, and brief duration—usually a few minutes, rarely over one hour—but during this time the patient is overwhelmed by fear and may believe they are going to die or go crazy. They may be exhausted after an attack.

2. *'Free-floating' anxiety* refers to a high level of anxiety that is more or less continuously present, is associated with physical symptoms (*see Table* 6.1) and has no obvious precipitants.

There may be discrete episodes of more severe anxiety or panic in addition.

3. *Phobic disorders* present rarely as emergencies except as a consequence of panic attacks in feared situations. Phobias are persistent and irrational fears that may be of specific objects (e.g. animals or hypodermic needles), specific situations (e.g. high places or dirt) or more generalised (e.g. fear of shops and crowded places in agoraphobia, or fear of social contact in social phobia). There is avoidance of the feared object or situation. The effect on the sufferer falls in the spectrum from negligible functional impairment to total disability.

4. *Obsessive compulsive illness* is also a far less common cause of emergency presentation than anxiety or panic attacks. Obsessions are recurrent, intrusive unwanted thoughts or impulses, and compulsions are repetitive ritualistic acts performed mechanically by the patient to ward off unpleasant consequences. Intense anxiety arises if the patient tries to resist either obsessional thoughts or compulsive acts.

One relatively common obsessional idea is that of the young mother who has the impulse to kill or injure her child. It is important to recognise this and differentiate it from the other causes of such thoughts (especially puerperal psychoses, depressive illness and poor self-control in personality disorders or drug abuse) as the patient with obsessional thoughts is able to resist them and can safely be reassured and sent home while urgent out-patient treatment is organised, whereas in other conditions the risk to the child can be grave.

5. *Other psychiatric disorders* may present with anxiety. Emotional distress may be a prominent feature of any psychiatric disorder. Symptoms of anxiety occuring as part of the illness are most common in depression, psychotic illnesses and organic brain syndromes. Symptoms of depression and anxiety commonly occur together.

## ASSESSMENT

Careful history taking and physical examination will usually distinguish anxiety states from physical illnesses presenting with anxiety, but problems may remain, especially with cardiac and pulmonary disease. Depending on the history and examination it may be useful to estimate arterial blood gases and obtain an electrocardiogram. Other possible tests include blood glucose and electrolytes, full blood count, urine drug screen, thyroid function tests and chest X-ray. Once organic disorders have been excluded then specific anxiety disorders can be considered.

It can be useful to distinguish so-called 'exogenous' anxiety felt in response to specific external events and situations from the anxiety disorders. To do this it is necessary to make a judgement about whether the degree of anxiety is appropriate to the level of stress. This can be very difficult, and when there is doubt then the patient's judgement should be respected.

Patients with anticipatory or situational anxiety can often be helped by being allowed to ventilate their fears, and by a practical counselling approach aimed at finding better ways of coping with difficult situations. Only rarely should they be treated pharmacologically, and then using single doses or very limited quantities. Predictable anxiety (for example, a patient who becomes excessively anxious on aeroplanes and has occasionally to fly abroad on business) may be helped by beta-blockers used shortly before the anxiety provoking event.

## EMERGENCY TREATMENT

The first priority is to control and reduce the level of anxiety. This must be followed by a definite treatment plan for the immediate future.

## CONTROLLING ANXIETY

The response of staff must be prompt; any delay will increase the patient's fears and intensify the demands for help. A firm, confident approach should be adopted. Staff should use the patient's name, introduce themselves and demonstrate that professional help is being offered. The patient should wait and be interviewed in a quiet room (preferably with space to pace up and down if needed). The assessment procedures and any treatment should be discussed with the patient and any relatives present, and the patient should be reminded of these plans at regular intervals.

Reassurance by word and deed is the mainstay of emergency treatment. The patient should be told his symptoms are caused by anxiety rather than serious physical illness. Being told that the symptoms are recognised as fitting a known pattern of illness provides the patient with a reason for previously unaccountable feelings.

Hyperventilation and its effects must be controlled. Talking with patients, getting them to become aware of and control their respiratory rate and depth or making them re-breathe into a paper bag held over the nose and mouth are useful techniques. Re-breathing can be dangerous in patients with respiratory distress and low blood oxygen and should only be done when cardiorespiratory causes for the symptoms have been excluded.

Simple relaxation techniques can help temporarily. The patient should be told to lie down, close his eyes, breathe slowly and relax various muscle groups in sequence. The staff member responsible must stay with the patient, giving quiet instruction, until the patient feels calmer. These techniques can be used at home by the patient.

Medication can be useful to control anxiety, but the patient must be told that this is a short-term measure to reduce symptoms, and that definitive treatment of the anxiety disorder will be instituted as quickly as possible. In general prescription of anti-anxiety medication is inadvisable, and should only be considered if the patient is in great and continuing distress.

If this course is adopted a short acting benzodiazepine is usually the the best choice (for example, lorazepam 1–2 mg). Parenteral administration is rarely necessary and carries the risk of respiratory depression. Continuing treatment with benzodiazepines for longer than seven days is inadvisable as tolerance rapidly develops and there is a serious danger of dependency. Prescriptions of longer duration or repeat prescriptions reduce the patient's chance of getting effective treatment.

Chronically anxious patients may present repeatedly, usually demanding medication to relieve their anxiety. This behaviour may evoke angry, rejecting or punitive responses from staff faced with these demands. General rules for dealing with such negative reactions are given elsewhere (q.v.), but one common response which should be avoided is to comply with the demand simply to get rid of the patient. This will increase dependency and reinforce the behaviour. Medication should only be offered as part of a broader treatment plan that is aimed at reducing both anxiety and consumption of drugs.

Patients presenting with phobias and obsessive-compulsive illnesses rarely require emergency treatment because their distress is chronic rather than acute. The offer of an early out-patient appointment with a psychiatrist or clinical psychologist will usually be sufficient to alleviate the immediate problem.

### FUTURE TREATMENT

Arranging follow-up is an important part of emergency treatment, as anxiety disorders are potentially treatable conditions that become more difficult to treat effectively the longer treatment is delayed. Referrals can be made to psychiatrists or directly to clinical psychologists if appro-

*Table* 6.3. TREATMENT STRATEGIES FOR ANXIETY-
RELATED DISORDERS

| Presenting syndrome | Treatment |
| --- | --- |
| Panic attacks | Antidepressants—tricyclics (imipramine), monoamine oxidase inhibitors (phenelzine) and trazodone—are all effective. Behavioural and psychotherapeutic techniques have little value. |
| Free floating anxiety | Imipramine can be effective in reducing anxiety. Beta-blockers reduce autonomic symptoms, but do not control psychological symptoms. Behavioural techniques (anxiety management) can be helpful. |
| Obsessional symptoms | Extremely difficult to treat. For obsessions antidepressants may be of some value. For compulsions a behavioural approach (response prevention) plus supportive psychotherapy should be tried. |
| Phobias | Behavioural treatment (graded exposure and practice) plus supportive psychotherapy. |

priate problems have been identified and delineated. General treatment strategies include pharmacotherapy, behavioural techniques and psychotherapy (*see Table* 6.3).

Antidepressant drugs have uncomfortable side-effects and are dangerous in overdose. They should only be prescribed for patients who are going to be followed up by the prescribing doctor. Anxious patients are often particularly sensitive to the side-effects of any medication, so possible side-effects should be explained and discussed before treatment is started. Medication should be initiated at low doses with only gradual increases.

# 7. Depression and dysphoria

Many patients present with complaints related to lowered mood. 'Depression' is a commonly used word reflecting a wide variety of experience from normal transient unhappiness to profoundly pathological states of hopelessness and negativism. It may be used to refer to anxiety, anger, grief, acute or chronic dysphoria and sometimes as an expression of the confusion and helplessness felt by dependent people whose support system has for some reason failed. The interviewer must explore the meaning of the complaint of depression in the patient's own terms.

## EMERGENCY PRESENTATION

Presentation as an emergency usually reflects a crisis or a change in functioning:

1. *Normal activity* may be disrupted—a patient may suddenly give up and stay in bed, or find himself unable to go to work or cope with normal daily responsibilities.
2. Many patients present following *suicide attempts* or episodes of deliberate self-harm. Still others request help because they are troubled by unwelcome but compelling *thoughts of suicide.*
3. They may complain of *physical symptoms* or others associated with depression without specifically mentioning lowered mood. Tiredness, insomnia and weight loss are typical worries.
4. Presentation may be *precipitated by others* who have become alarmed at the change in the patient or his behaviour, or who have become angry, hopeless or rejecting because of the patient's continuing black mood and apparent helplessness.

5. The patient's *attempts to cope* with the depression may directly cause the presentation, for example intoxication with alcohol or drugs.
6. Finally some patients will complain specifically of *depressed mood* experienced as abnormal for them.

Depression and elation can be normal conditions, are a component of many psychiatric syndromes or may be secondary to physical illness. Most psychiatric illnesses can be associated with secondary depression and virtually any medical illness can cause depression. Some of the more common ones are given in *Table* 7.1, although this is far from an exhaustive list.

*Table* 7.1. ORGANIC CAUSES OF DEPRESSION

| Cause | Examples |
|---|---|
| Infections | Influenza; mononucleosis |
| Drugs | Antihypertensives; steroids; alcohol |
| Endocrine disorders | Hypothyroidism; Cushing's syndrome |
| Neurological illness | Parkinson's disease; MS; CVA |
| Malignant diseases | Carcinoma of lung; brain tumours |
| Drug withdrawal | Amphetamines |

## CLASSIFICATION OF DEPRESSION

Attempts to classify depressive syndromes have proved difficult and are clinically of little practical value. A descriptive approach to the patient's symptoms and signs is probably more valuable. Distinctions such as those between 'reactive' and 'endogenous' or between 'neurotic' and 'psychotic' depressive illnesses have little clinical application. The classification used here is based on DSM-III, but is a clinical classification. The depressive syndromes are distinguished by their severity. In general depressive episodes occurring in recurrent depressive illness and those in bipolar (manic-depressive) illnesses do not differ in their course or response to treatment.

## 1. MAJOR DEPRESSIVE EPISODES

For the diagnosis of a *major depressive episode* DSM-III requires that the patient suffers from low mood for at least two weeks in the presence of at least four of: appetite disturbance (particulary lowered appetite with weight loss); sleep disturbance (particulary waking early in the morning); psychomotor retardation or agitation; loss of pleasure or enjoyment (anhedonia); loss of energy; feelings of guilt or worthlessness; poor memory or concentration; suicidal thoughts. This represents a *moderate* severity of depression.

History and mental state examination reveal a number of other features:

a. The patient's *appearance* may show signs of self-neglect. He may look depressed and miserable, sitting with hunched shoulders and downward gaze. Depressed patients may be able to smile appropriately, but this is unlikely to be consistent. Movement may be slow and retarded, or occasionally there will be agitation, with fidgeting, picking at clothing and hand-wringing.

b. His *mood* is of all-pervading misery which does not change significantly in response to his surroundings. There may also be anxiety or irritability.

c. *Thoughts* will be pessimistic or hopeless. The patient may believe he is failing at work or as a family man. He will see the future as hopeless, his life as not worth living and he may have contemplated suicide. He may have gloomy memories or excessive guilt about minor transgressions in the distant past.

d. *Physical symptoms* may be prominent, for example generalised pain and discomfort. The patient may be preoccupied with hypochondriacal ideas.
e. *Psychological symptoms* include poor memory and concentration, preoccupying or even obsessional thoughts, brooding to the extent of neglecting work or normal occupations and phobic symptoms.

## 2. MAJOR DEPRESSIVE EPISODES WITH PSYCHOTIC FEATURES

These represent a significantly greater degree of severity in the spectrum of depressive illnesses. All the above symptoms will be present, perhaps with added intensity, and in addition the patient displays poor judgement and loses the ability correctly to assess the reality of his experience. Characteristic features include:

a. *Delusions* of worthlessness or guilt, of being justifiably persecuted or punished, of ill-health or poverty and ruin.
b. There may be *auditory hallucinations*, often of accusing or critical voices.
c. In *Cotard's syndrome* there are 'nihilistic delusions', such as the patient's intestines having rotted away, the patient and his family being dead, or the whole world being in a state of decay.
d. There may be severe degrees of *agitation*, especially in older patients, or of *psychomotor retardation* that can be so severe that the patient is stuporose.

The risk of suicide in these severe depressions is very high, and patients presenting in this way require urgent hospitalisation.

## 3. DYSTHYMIC DISORDER

This category represents the DSM-III equivalent of neurotic depression and depressive personality and covers the *mild* category of depressive illness. The patient experiences depressed mood but other symptoms, especially the 'biological' symptoms (appetite and sleep disturbance, lowered libido, reduced energy) are not present. The criteria for a major depressive episode are not met.

In DSM-III dysthymic disorder has to be chronic, lasting at least two years, but in practice similar symptoms of shorter duration are often seen, for example in cases of deliberate self-poisoning (q.v.). These would be classified as adjustment reactions, but treatment is effectively the same. There may be some degree of impairment in social functioning, especially if the symptoms are of long duration. These patients often present in psychosocial crisis or with the complications of drug or alcohol abuse (q.v.).

The importance of distinguishing these patients from those suffering from major depressive episodes is that dysthymic disorders generally respond very poorly to antidepressant medication, which should therefore be used with great reluctance.

## 4. GRIEF

Grief is an adaptive response to the experience of loss. Mourning can mimic depression, but self-esteem is not lost, the focus of the patient's ruminations is the lost person or object, the patient has hope for the future and often sees the process of mourning as positive. The interviewer's role is to facilitate the process of mourning. Psychotropic medication is not indicated.

The depressive syndromes outlined above need to be differentiated from normal sadness, anxiety states (q.v.), obsessional or phobic disorders, schizophrenia and dementia, all of which can present with low mood. In some cases of apparent dementia the loss of cognitive function is itself a symptom of depression ('depressive pseudodementia'—q.v.) and is reversible when the depression is treated.

## PRECIPITATING FACTORS IN DEPRESSION

There has been much interest recently in the role of recent life events in the causation of depressive illnesses. The frequency of life events is raised in the months before depression, but this is in general true for all psychiatric illnesses and for deliberate self-harm (q.v.), in which there need be no psychiatric illness present. Life events involving some form of loss have been associated with depression, but only some 10% of people suffering loss events become depressed. In addition life events could be the consequence of the developing illness, or be retrospectively seen as causal by the patient, or even be coincidental.

The presence or absence of life events in the recent past of depressed patients may help in understanding their predicament, but has no significance for treatment. Depressive illnesses with no apparent precipitants are not necessarily more severe illnesses, nor does the fact that depression is 'understandable' make it less amenable to physical treatment.

## ASSESSMENT

An adequate history covering all the areas outlined above is essential. The history should include use of prescribed and non-prescribed drugs, evidence of excessive alcohol use, any previous psychiatric history and a full mental state examination. A careful medical history and physical examination should be considered essential. All depressed patients must be assessed very carefully for risk of suicide (q.v.).

Once the diagnosis has been established, treatment will need to be based on an assessment of the patient's resources:

1. *External:*
    —previous response to drugs or other treatment;
    —friends, family and social support available;

—current or recent psychiatric care and how quickly the patient can be seen;

—the reasons for and response to previous admissions, if psychiatric admission is being considered.

2. *Internal:*

—the patient's understanding of his symptoms. Does he see them as illness, or does he believe he is worthless?

—the patient's trust in medical treatment and optimism about the outcome of treatment;

—impulse control, particularly resistance to suicidal ideas or impulses;

—the patient's experience of previous episodes, and his expectations of treatment.

Even with this information, decisions about depressed patients are always to some extent a matter of personal judgement, and there will always be risks. A good rule is always to err on the side of safety.

*Case example:* A 50-year-old man was referred to psychiatric out-patients for an urgent assessment of his depression. He clearly had a major depressive illness of some severity, including suicidal ideas. However, he denied any suicidal plans or intent, saying that he could never harm himself for the sake of his family. His wife and daughter were also present at the interview, and felt that the patient would not succumb to suicidal impulses. The patient refused admission, supported by his relatives, but accepted a prescription for one week's supply of antidepressants and a further appointment in one week's time. The day of his appointment he woke early, felt unbearably that life was not worth living and attempted suicide by cutting his throat. Fortunately he survived, and made a full recovery after appropriate in-patient treatment.

## TREATMENT

An organised, effective approach counters the patient's attitude of helplessness and hopelessness. It is important to avoid getting angry (for example, if the patient refuses treatment because he feels unworthy, or is too pessimistic to believe it will work) or impatient with slowness or repetitiveness. While the patient is not being interviewed a member of staff or a relative should stay with the patient.

## 1. PSYCHOLOGICAL TREATMENT (INCLUDING INSTILLATION OF HOPE)

a. *Empathic exploration* of the patient's feelings and current problems, paying special attention to psychosocial factors that could have precipitated the depression, help the patient feel understood, and establish a firm basis for compliance with treatment.

b. *Reframing the symptoms* as a psychiatric diagnosis ('your low mood, poor appetite, lack of energy and difficulty concentrating add up to a kind of illness that we call depression, and I'd like to talk about how we treat that') helps the patient understand his problems in a new way that implies he is ill rather than, for example, wicked and deserving of his misery.

c. The interviewer must adopt an *optimistic stance to treatment,* offering expected positive effects, and including a clear statement of the reasons for treatment being necessary.

d. Many acute problems will be amenable to a *crisis intervention approach* (q.v.), which can be used in isolation or as an adjunct to psychotropic medication.

## 2. MEDICATION

The treatment of choice for major depressive illnesses is antidepressant drugs, but the slow onset of improvement, distressing and sometimes dangerous side-effects and the risk of overdose mean that only doctors prepared to take responsibility for follow-up and careful supervision of treatment should give the first prescription.

Poor compliance with antidepressant medication is common. This can be minimised by:

a. *Explaining the nature and effects* of treatment (including the slow onset of therapeutic effect, the duration of treatment and the necessity to take the tablets as prescribed).

b. *Describing and discussing the side-effects* that can be expected.

c. *Starting at a low dose* and gradually increasing to minimise side-effects.

d. *Asking if the patient has any questions or worries.*

Early follow-up will be required, so the patient need only be prescribed a limited number of tablets to reduce the risk from a possible overdose. If need be this measure should be discussed openly with the patient ('Sometimes when people get depressed they get so low they feel like harming themselves—how would you feel if I only gave you a few days supply of tablets to start with?').

Other effective treatments for depression such as lithium, electroconvulsive therapy (ECT) and neuroleptics (for agitation or psychotic features) should only be given after a specialist opinion has been obtained. Monoamine oxidase inhibitors (MAOIs) are effective antidepressants, but the dietary restrictions and potential risks make it inadvisable to prescribe these as a first-line treatment in preference to other antidepressants.

## 3. FOLLOW-UP

As a general rule, if low mood, or minor disturbance of sleep, appetite or energy, dominate the clinical picture, then psychosocial measures should be the first line of treatment. If there are more severe symptoms such as loss of concentration, loss of interest and enjoyment, early morning wakening and diurnal variation of mood then psychotropic medication should be considered in addition. If the patient expresses feelings of hopelessness or life not being worth living, is experiencing guilt and self-blame or feelings of worthlessness and suicidal ideas then a very careful assessment is essential and urgent referral to a psychiatrist should be considered. The patient should not be sent away if there is doubt about the diagnosis or the severity of the depression.

*Psychiatric admission* may be necessary if:

a. psychotic features are present;
b. there is a high suicide risk;
c. social support is absent or inadequate;
d. the patient needs intensive nursing care;
c. there is doubt about the severity of the depression.

If out-patient care is thought to be most appropriate then the emergency clinician must accept responsibility for arranging adequate follow-up care. Good communication with the patient's general practitioner or the psychiatric out-patient department is necessary to obtain an early appointment. If possible these arrangements should be made before the patient leaves. Any arrangements about follow-up must be clearly communicated to the patient and to any relatives or friends present, and they should be made clear about how to get urgent help should the need arise.

With treatment the average duration of a depressive episode is 3 months, and remission is common between episodes. However, recurrence is very likely and between 11% and 17% of patients with a depressive disorder will eventually commit suicide.

# 8. Patients with abnormal personalities

Personality describes the characteristic attitudes, behaviours and emotional responses which make a person distinctive. It is manifest in the ways in which a person interacts with his environment and relates to others. To be described as features of personality these characteristics must be consistent over time, usually appearing in adolescence, and are distinct from changes in function caused by illness.

If these characteristics consistently cause significant impairment in social or occupational functioning or subjective distress then the patient may be said to have a personality disorder.

The most common presentations are:

1. Depressed mood, often with suicidal ideation or deliberate self-harm.
2. Anxiety and increasing social disorganisation.
3. Escalation of impulsive or harmful behaviour, for example drug and alcohol abuse, or apparently uncontrollable emotions such as rage. These patients are usually brought by another person who is worried or fearful.

A common request is for medication to control dysphoric mood or impulsive behaviour.

## DIAGNOSIS

Unfortunately diagnostic classifications of personality disorder (the American DSM-III manual describes 12 distinct types) are imprecise, and overlap between symptoms renders the distinctions clinically unhelpful.

Patients who fit the concept of personality disorder usually fall into one of three categories (modified from Campbell and Russell, 1983):

1. Emotional instability, angry, impulsive, seductive or over-dramatic behaviour, associated with a history of at least one of the following:
   —recurrent failures and conflict in relationships;
   —recurrent episodes of impulsive or aggressive behaviour;
   —frequent changes of employment;
   —frequent contacts with the law or conflict with authority;
   —multiple drug abuse;
   —repeated self-injury or overdoses;
   —long-standing instability of mood.
2. Odd, isolated, sensitive, suspicious or eccentric behaviour associated with evidence of long-standing excessive introspection and aloofness.
3. Fearful, helpless or dependent behaviour with a history of:
   —marked overdependence on others;
   —repeated investigations of unexplained physical symptoms;
   —recurrent behavioural disorder or neurotic symptoms in response to normal life stress.

The personality disorders most commonly seen as emergencies are those in group 1—the so-called histrionic or antisocial personalities. They must be differentiated from organic brain syndromes, acute or chronic psychoses, and drug or alcohol abuse (q.v.). Patients with physical symptoms or repeated stress reactions may be found on medical wards, in general practice or presenting to many other agencies. The most common mistake in such patients is to misdiagnose them as neurotic and treat them symptomatically for anxiety or depression.

Difficulties in diagnosis may arise because of the brief time available in emergency settings and the substantial amount of historical information that has to be obtained to establish characteristic personality patterns. In addition there is a danger in diagnosing a person too rapidly as personality disordered and missing other disorders such as drug and alcohol abuse, functional illnesses (e.g. depression or psychosis) or medical illnesses (e.g. subdural haemorrhage or delirium). Any patient with self-damaging behaviour or ideation should be assessed for the risk of suicide (q.v.).

Both the feelings and behaviour of personality disordered patients pose difficulties for staff. Mood is usually intense and 'contagious' and may be anger, depression, boredom, emptiness or helplessness. Behaviours are impulsive and may be self-destructive impulses: drug abuse, chaotic sexuality, eating disorders, self-mutilation or suicide atttempts.

A diagnosis of personality disorder tends to carry negative connotations, including a belief that the patient's distress or complaints need not be taken seriously. Epithets such as 'attention–seeking', 'manipulative' and 'immature' are used to justify too ready dismissal. As with all emergency presentations no patient should be sent away without a full assessment being completed, some degree of understanding of why the patient should present in this way and at this time being gained, and an attempt made to help resolve the crisis.

## ASSESSMENT

All patients require rapid but thorough assessment. Particular problems arise with patients felt to be potentially violent or dangerous and approaches to these patients are covered in Chapter 10. The strong emotional responses personality disordered patients usually arouse in others can put them into the category of 'difficult patients', and techniques for dealing with the difficulties that arise are also covered elsewhere (see Chapter 3).

Patients may not recognise problems in their personality, or give ill-focussed or rambling histories. In these cases it is essential to obtain information from another informant. Old notes, if available, can provide valuable historical information and allow changes to be more readily detected. Other involved services or agencies can often provide valuable advice or information over the telephone.

*APPROACHING THE PATIENT*

The label personality disorder is often associated with the belief that there is no treatment and therefore intervention is pointless. As a consequence the patient is dismissed with a label such as 'hysterical' or 'psychopathic' and no attempt is made to understand him in terms of his individual strengths and weaknesses. The most important part of the interview is to understand the current crisis and how the patient's normal level of adjustment is disturbed. Events leading up to presentation should be explored and related to what is known about the patient's history, especially similar occurrences in the past.

If the patient is vague or rambling, the interview must be stuctured and focussed. Many patients will not volunteer information about important areas such as drug abuse or court convictions unless they are asked directly.

Special attention should be paid to:

1. Available social support:
   —How is it disrupted by the current crisis?
   —How have similar crises been dealt with before?
   —Is there sufficient support (physical, financial, emotional, etc.) available to cope with the current difficulties?
2. Is the patient currently in psychiatric care?
   —What does this involve?
   —Have there been any changes or problems in

treatment (for example, recent or threatened discharge)?
—Does the patient have unrealistic expectations of treatment?
3. Is there any evidence of an underlying functional or medical disorder?
4. Family factors:
—Do the family understand and support any current treatment programme?
—What role does the patient's behaviour play in the family (e.g. controlling others)?
—Is the patient's family itself disorganised or chaotic?
—Are family members over-involved with the patient and his behaviour?

## MANAGEMENT

### GENERAL ISSUES

Patients with personality disorders can be amongst the most difficult patients to assess and treat. The interviewer is frequently left feeling frustrated, puzzled or angry, and may get caught up in the patient's maladaptive ways of relating to others. For instance, impulsive or aggressive patients readily provoke angry and rejecting responses, whereas dependent patients draw others into feeling responsible for them.

The interviewer can recognise such unhelpful emotional involvement by the powerful but confusing feelings such patients arouse. Having only positive feelings for patients is not a prerequisite for effective treatment, but denying or ignoring negative and uncomfortable feelings can lead the unwary into missing a valuable clue to the underlying problem, as well as hindering treatment. The patient's maladaptive behaviour is *not* calculated, but an enduring difficulty he feels unable to control. The interviewer should recognise its habitual qualities and not take it personally, but instead focus on the physical or emotional complaints of the patient in a supportive and non-judgmental way.

## PSYCHIATRIC TREATMENT

Many patients with disordered personalities will not request psychiatric help or recognise problems relating to their personality structure. Any treatment for the personality disorder will be prolonged and require careful planning. Treatment should instead focus on treating associated physical illness or psychiatric illness and addressing the current crisis and its resolution, using crisis intervention techniques (q.v.).

Often the patient and physician will be at odds, for example if the patient is demanding sedative drugs inappropriately. In such cases it is best to be honest about the dilemma and try to enlist the patient's own strengths in finding a solution ('You say you won't sleep at all unless I give you these tablets, but I believe they're harmful for you. Do you think you could manage to cope just for a day or two until I can get in touch with the doctor you normally see in the clinic and ask him to see you?'). If members of the patient's family or others are with the patient they should be involved in these discussions. Helping them understand the nature of the current crisis can help them organise their own coping skills more effectively.

## DRUG TREATMENT

Medication is rarely indicated for patients with personality disorders presenting in crisis. If specific treatments seem indicated, for example antidepressants, it is best to reassess the patient at a follow-up visit, as mood states are often fluctuating and the pattern of the crisis might well become clearer. As a general rule no prescriptions should be issued for drugs carrying a risk of dependence, especially methadone or benzodiazepines. Some patients will be clearly dependent on prescribed drugs, especially bensodiazepines, but in these cases no more than a 48-hours supply should be given, on the clear understanding that arrangements will be made for follow-up aimed at reducing the dependence.

## HOSPITAL ADMISSION

Patients should be encouraged to accept as much responsibility as they can, so admission should be avoided wherever possible. However, some patients will present with problems severe enough to warrant admission. For example:

1. If there is a high risk of suicide (q.v.).
2. If there is evidence that the patient's behaviour constitutes a risk to themselves and others (although *see* Chapter 10 on the management of violent behaviour).
3. If the patient's social support systems have entirely broken down.
4. If there is an associated illness requiring admission (e.g. severe depression).

Arrangements for admission should involve careful consultation and discussion with the admitting psychiatrist, with a positive aim for treatment, not merely to relieve staff difficulties. If may be necessary to admit patients involuntarily, for example if there is a high risk of suicide.

# 9. Psychiatric presentations of neurological illness: catatonic, mute and stuporose patients

Among the important medical conditions that can be missed by a too eager attempt to ascribe symptoms to psychiatric illness are a number of neurological conditions. Common neurological conditions that can present with psychiatric symptoms are listed in *Table* 9.1. This table, with much else in this chapter, is based on Lishman's (1978) definitive textbook of organic psychiatry.

Epilepsy may be associated with psychological symptoms in the pre-ictal, ictal or post-ictal periods (*see Table* 9.2).

The possibility of neurological or medical disorder should be thoroughly investigated if:

1. The history indicates a relatively sudden onset of psychiatric symptoms with no previous psychiatric history.
2. There is a history of fluctuating or intermittent psychiatric symptomatology.
3. There is any evidence of clouding of consciousness.
4. The mental state findings are atypical of recognised psychiatric illness.
5. There is a history of recent medical or neurological illness, especially with fluctuating symptoms.
6. There is a history of head injury.
7. There is no evidence of drug or alcohol abuse.

In addition to mental state examination (q.v.) the patient will require thorough neurological examination, including level of consciousness, cognitive abilities, the presence of so-

*Table* 9.1. NEUROLOGICAL ILLNESSES THAT CAN PRESENT
WITH PSYCHIATRIC SYMPTOMS

| *Illness* | *Psychiatric symptom* |
| --- | --- |
| Cerebrovascular disease | Depression<br>Personality changes<br>Variable amnesia<br>Transient confusion<br>Schizophrenia-like psychosis |
| Parkinson's disease | Depression<br>Confusional states<br>Cognitive impairment |
| CNS infections | Schizophrenia-like psychosis<br>Hallucinations<br>Depression or elation<br>Personality changes<br>Aggressiveness and impaired judgement<br>Mutism |
| Narcolepsy<br>Multiple sclerosis<br>Myaesthenia gravis<br>Cerebrovascular disease | Mutiple or transient symptoms may mimic<br>  hysteria |
| Huntington's chorea<br>  (very rare) | Paranoia<br>Personality changes<br>Affective changes (mania or depression)<br>Hallucinations or delusions<br>Suicide |
| Wilson's disease<br>  (very rare) | Argumentativeness<br>Labile mood<br>Cognitive impairment<br>Depression |

called 'soft' neurological signs (hesitant speech, mild dysarthria, restlessness, hypokinesia, clumsiness, poor balance,
poor coordination) and signs of the emergence of primitive
reflexes (grasp, sucking, snout, palmomental or glabellar
tap).

*Table* 9.2. PSYCHIATRIC SYMPTOMS IN EPILEPSY

| | |
|---|---|
| Pre-ictal (aura) | Unusual sensations (epigastric or elsewhere)<br>Hallucinatory phenomena (e.g. acrid smells) |
| Ictal (complex-<br>partial seizures) | Hallucinations (visual, aural, taste, smell)<br>Automatisms<br>Loose associations<br>Delusions of persecution or thought control<br>Rage attacks<br>Dissociative states |
| Petit mal seizures | Stupor<br>Absences |
| Post-ictal | Reduced level of consciousness<br>Mood changes<br>Rambling speech or dysphasia<br>Paranoid, hallucinatory states (may endure)<br>Disorientation<br>Restlessness, irritability<br>Incoherence |

As well as the special investigations needed to exclude organic causes of psychiatric illness (q.v.), if neurological disease is suspected the patient may require a lumbar puncture, electroencephalography and a computerised tomographic brain scan.

If there is any doubt about aetiology the patient should be admitted to a medical or neurological ward for full investigation.


## STUPOR

Stuporose patients are mute and immobile but seem to be conscious by the fact they demonstrate purposeful eye movements, or register (by blinking, etc.) painful stimuli without withdrawing. About 20% of stupors have an

*Table* 9.3. THE CAUSES OF STUPOR

| | |
|---|---|
| Psychiatric | Schizophrenia<br>Psychotic depression<br>Hysteria<br>Feigned psychosis<br>Neuroleptic medication |
| Intoxication | Alcohol<br>Hallucinogenic drugs |
| Neurological | Focal lesions of the brain stem, limbic system, frontal<br>   or temporal lobes<br>Encephalitis<br>Epilepsy (e.g. petit mal status)<br>Parkinson's disease |
| Metabolic | Hypoglycaemia<br>Hypercalcaemia<br>Acute intermittent porphyria<br>Uraemia<br>Hepatic encephalopathy |

organic cause (*see Table* 9.3), and it can be very difficult to distinguish organic from functional stupors. Thus on first presentation stupor should be considered a medical emergency.

There may be classical catatonic features—waxy flexibility, automatic obedience to commands and negativistic resistance to passive movement—in both organic and functional stupors. The best distinguishing feature is a history of psychiatric illness with similar presentation. Patients in depressive stupor may present a very depressed facial appearance. Functional stupors may fluctuate or improve; organic stupors tend to worsen.

EEG recording will show a normal waking state in hysteria or patients feigning illness and will be grossly abnormal in toxic states, brain-stem lesions or encephalitis. Focal abnormalities could be demonstrated, and the typical pattern of spikes and waves in epileptic status may be seen.

Stuporose patients can become severely dehydrated and may need intravenous or nasogastric feeding. Once organic causes have been ruled out, patients with functional stupor generally recover rapidly following a single application of electroconvulsive therapy.

## MUTISM

Mutism not associated with stupor is rare. The patient with hysterical mutism or aphonia has total loss of vocalisation with no structural abnormalities and normal coughing. If there is evidence of phonation (normal coughing or other vocal noises) with no speech, then in most cases no intervention other then reassurance is required. There are usually other features suggestive of hysteria, and treatment strategies are similar to other hysterical conversion disorders (q.v.).

# Part C
# Situations posing special difficulties

# 10. Dealing with anger, aggression and violence

The emotional state usually associated with aggression (defined as verbal or physical attack) is *anger*, because that is commonly our own experience when we are aware of being aggressive. However, aggression may arise from feelings of *despair* or *frustration* which may not all be consciously perceived as containing hostile elements, although often careful questioning will elicit these. *Low self-esteem* or a sense of *humiliation* may be a potent factor in triggering aggression.

*Case example:* A consultant ordered a 17-year-old attending the casualty department with an infected tattoo to take the chewing gum out of his mouth. The effects of this encounter may well have rebounded on the colleague who some days later revived memories of this event by rather casual instructions to the patient, precipitating an aggressive verbal response, somewhat disinhibited by alcohol, in the patient.

When defined widely, as above, aggression can be viewed as a normal and understandable part of man's behaviour. The mentally ill are in general no more likely to be violent than other members of the public and serious violence associated with psychiatric illness is rare. Intoxication with alcohol or other drugs is probably the commonest contributory factor to violence anywhere.

## ANGER AS A NORMAL EMOTION

Anger is often experienced as justified by the angry person, but is rarely experienced that way by others. Angry outbursts usually fade gradually leaving the individual feeling annoyed with himself, and therefore vulnerable to comments or attitudes which do not allow the regaining of composure without loss of face. The aim in dealing with anger should be to avoid the stimulation of aggressive reflexes by confrontation and to assist the angry patient to turn his feelings into thought and verbal expression.

Anger may be expressed in many ways. As in all diagnosis the history is of primary importance.

*Case example:* A 61-year-old man with carcinoma of the bronchus was referred for a psychiatric opinion. This was his second admission after radiotherapy, and he appeared angry and withdrawn. The referral queried whether he was depressed. After his first radiotherapy he had a productive cough at night, and used his chamber pot as a receptacle for sputum. The next morning he was distressed to find the pot full of bloody debris. On telephoning the hospital he was told this was normal following radiotherapy. He wrongly got the impression that staff felt his worry was not sufficiently important to bother the hospital. The psychiatrist's impression was that he was very angry following his frightening experience and cavalier dismissal, with resulting loss of confidence in the staff. He was further angered by the lack of understanding demonstrated by the referral to a psychiatrist.

The referral had correctly described his symptoms, but there had not been time allowed to enable him to talk about how he felt and why. It would take some time for him to relate well to the ward again, and the experience may well have affected his compliance with essential treatment. The task of resolving these feelings is the responsibility of the ward staff and it would not be appropriate for a psychiatrist to be involved further with the patient.

This is an example of normal anger and also illustrates some aspects of dealing with disturbance which are covered more fully in the section on referral to a psychiatrist (q.v.)

## MORBID ANGER

Morbidity in the psychiatric sense usually implies an intensity and/or duration of a symptom which is out of proportion to the stimulus and interferes significantly with normal living. In morbid jealousy (q.v.), for example, seething anger towards a spouse's real or imagined infidelity may dominate the aggrieved partner's life so that work is given up and elaborate surveillance instigated.

There are several categories of psychiatric illness that can produce anger, loss of self-control and possible violence. A brief list is included for completeness. Assessment and management of these conditions are covered in the appropriate chapters.

1. Psychosis:
   —acute paranoid psychosis
   —hypomania
   —morbid jealousy
2. Acute organic brain syndromes (delirium)
3. Drugs:
   —intoxication (all sedative drugs, amphetamine, solvents)
   —withdrawal (esp. opiates, sedative drugs)
   —attempts to obtain supplies
4. Neurological disease:
   —head injury (recent or remote)
   —chronic organic syndromes
   —epilepsy
5. Personality disorder

## VIOLENCE CAN OCCUR ANYWHERE

### 1. THE ACCIDENT AND EMERGENCY DEPARTMENT (INCLUDING THE EMERGENCY PSYCHIATRIC CLINIC)

Violence in this department often presents considerable difficulty as the individual involved is often unknown and there are no independent informants as to the nature of the problem. Commonly the risk of violence is identified by someone other than the patient, who is brought to hospital by others, often police or relatives. He may already have been confronted in an argumentative fashion, or handled roughly and if so will be angry and suspicious.

## 2. THE PSYCHIATRIC WARD

Many staff in psychiatric units are likely to have had some experience of dealing with violent incidents but few units are well staffed, especially at night. Often if a new, potentially violent, patient is to be admitted there will be time to arrange for optimum cover with senior nursing staff involved from the earliest stages of the proposed admission. It is important that the admitting medical officer responds more by his presence than by liberal prescription of tranquillisers once admission has been achieved and that the approach to aggression acknowledges the normal feelings towards a (possibly involuntary) admission as well as those related to the acute illness.

## 3. THE GENERAL MEDICAL OR SURGICAL WARD

The casualty department and perhaps the acute psychiatric ward bear the brunt of aggressive behaviour and to some extent bear this philosophically, or at least accept the inevitability of some violent incidents. General wards, where such incidents are rarer, may be less tolerant of behaviour seen to be awkward or out of place. For this reason a systematic way of approaching anger and aggression is of considerable help.

## ASSESSMENT

In dealing with the threat of violence, making a clinical diagnosis is rarely a primary consideration, as the urgent response tends to be similar whatever the formal diagnosis. Adequate examination cannot take place until anger and aggression has been contained, but then it is essential to remember the possible pitfalls in the A & E department—

alcohol masking injuries sustained in fights and falls by its anaesthetic effect, or contributing to a confusional state following head injury. Hypoglycaemia and epilepsy should always be considered (*see* Chapter 5).

## PRINCIPLES OF DEALING WITH ANGER AND AGGRESSION

Aggression in the hospital setting is likely to provoke aggressive responses in staff which cause premature judgements to be made.

It is a good idea to be prepared in advance. If possible review old notes and talk to independent informants to gain some sense of the nature of the problem. If the interviewer feels unable to cope he is likely to become angry himself—this will quickly be detected by the patient and complicate the situation.

A simple but systematic approach can be invaluable, and guidelines for assessment are given in *Table* 10.1. Three general principles should always be followed:

1. The patient should always be treated rationally.
2. Control should be established early.
3. Challenging confrontations should be avoided.

*Case example:* A patient with an acute psychotic illness was insisting on leaving the ward and had threatened the nurses and broken a window when asked to remain. The nursing officer requested that four male nurses from other wards came to give support. When the extra nurses arrived, three stayed just outside the ward, while the other stood quietly in the corridor by the patient's room. The duty psychiatrist went alone into the patient's room, leaving the door open. After introducing himself and explaining why he had been called to the ward he asked the cause of the patient's obvious anger. He responded to the patient's repeated insistence on leaving by stating clearly that he had a duty to detain the patient if he tried to leave in his current mood, and was prepared to do so. The patient was also allowed to understand that sufficient staff were available to

*Table* 10.1. GUIDELINES FOR ASSESSING A POTENTIALLY VIOLENT PATIENT

---

*The patient:*
1. The interviewer should clearly be concerned for the patient's best interests, even if he and the patient disagree about what those best interests are.
2. Interviews should be leisurely and not smack of interrogation.
3. The interviewer should introduce himself, and clearly state his desire to understand what is going on.
4. The purpose of the interview, and any action which is taken, should be explained clearly to the patient at all stages.
5. The patient should not be challenged or confronted. Reflect the anger back calmly to the patient to explore its meaning. Listen to all fears and grievances: Has the aggressive behaviour any meaning to the patient? Are there any provoking factors which can be removed?
6. No comment should be made on the patient's personality or other characteristics, either verbally or by attitude.
7. Allow the patient the opportunity to withdraw from confrontation without losing face.

*The setting:*
1. It is usually preferable to interview the patient alone, but within calling distance of other staff.
2. The interview should be in a quiet setting. Dealing with an angry patient in a hospital corridor or a noisy office is likely to provoke fear and hostility in others.
3. Sitting down is less threatening than standing.
4. If there are signs during the interview that the patient is unable to maintain control, such as increasing restlessness or threats, then the interviewer should emphasise that he is prepared to assist by using external controls.
5. Discussion with other members of staff is best continued out of line of sight of the patient. An angry suspicious patient may incorrectly interpret smiles or whispered asides or misinterpret similar actions not related to him.
6. The interview should not be completed until the problem is defined and arrangements for future care have been made.

---

support this promise. The patient agreed to stay, but remained angry. He began to complain about excess medication making him drowsy and having adverse side-effects. Although the doctor refused to reduce the total daily dosage prescribed by the patient's consultant he was able to offer a change in the way the drug was given so that a larger amount was taken at night and proportionally less in the daytime. The patient was satisfied with this compromise and agreed to stay on the ward on a voluntary basis.

Warning signals of potential violence include:
1. Verbal warning from the patient or his escorts.
2. Marked restlessness.
3. Bruising or signs of injury, including self-injury.
4. Needle tracks or other signs of drug abuse.
5. Staff intuition or apprehension.
6. A past history of impulsive or seriously irresponsible behaviour.

Enquiry should be made about the patient's temper; any history of fighting, perhaps involving the police or courts; any reckless behaviour such as dangerous driving or frequent drunkenness. Evidence of violence in the family of origin is significantly related to aggression in adult life.

The interviewer should attempt to obtain some idea of how well established the threat of violence might be:

1. Has the patient made any concrete plans for carrying out his threat?
2. Are the means for carrying it out readily available?
3. Are the plans realistic?
4. Is there evidence of any previous attack?

An open threat of violence is often related to fear of loss of control and can be seen as a request for help. Veiled threats or hints can be more sinister and should always be followed up during interview. If the threat is towards a named person or persons then this should be taken very seriously and the patient's relationship with the proposed victims explored.

Such threats may be part of a delusional system or part of a paranoid, jealous rage such as in the syndrome of morbid jealousy (q.v.). In some cases aggression or violence may have been part of a relationship for years. Sometimes a threat may be reported by others but denied by the patient, in which case it can be informative to include the proposed victim in a joint interview which may clarify the relationship or uncover hidden rage or impending loss of control.

An attempt should be made to determine whether the patient is carrying a weapon at the time of the interview. If so then it is not advisable to demand that it be handed over immediately. A sympathetic approach after the issues have been discussed, along the lines of 'It would be a shame if anyone got hurt while you are so upset, so why don't you let me keep that for you?', is more likely to achieve the desired result. If the patient remains uncooperative, or if physical restraint becomes imperative then the police should be involved. No one should be allowed to retain possession of a dangerous weapon in a hospital or clinic.

## WHEN TO INVOLVE THE POLICE

If threatened or actual violence persists then the patient should be told that the police will be called if required. In rare extreme cases it may in the end prove necessary to request assistance from the police. Sometimes a policeman or security officer just standing where he can be seen can calm undue excitement.

In the very rare cases where these guidelines are insufficient to contain the situation then it will probably be necessary to utilise external controls by restraint or medication. This should not be seen as a retaliatory or punitive measure but simply as temporary help until the patient is able to regain control of himself. Restraint should usually be necessary only when there is a serious risk of injury to the patient or others by assault or as a consequence of damage to property.

## WHEN TO USE FORCE

To avoid an uncoordinated, undignified and possibly dangerous struggle:

1. Potentially violent patients should be kept under observation until such time as the risk of violence can be excluded.
2. Staff involved should be calm and behave as unobtrusively as possible.
3. The patient should not feel they have to prove something, which can be achieved by having enough staff to make any fight 'no contest'.
4. Any action should be planned in advance, with each person's role being made clear, and should preferably be undertaken only by staff with experience in such situations.

The degree of force used must be the minimum required to control the patient. However, it is likely that several staff members acting together can subdue an aggressive patient with less force than one or two who might have to struggle.

### USE OF PHYSICAL RESTRAINT

1. The first aim is to cause no injury to anyone involved.
2. Begin by pinning the patient's arms to his body from behind.
3. From this position it is usually possible to bring the patient to the ground and have someone lie across his legs.
4. Pressure should never be applied to the neck, chest or abdomen as this can severely limit respiration or cause injury to vulnerable areas. Panic from fear of suffocation will lead to understandably fierce resistance to restraint.
5. If arms or legs are held this should be close to major joints to avoid the risk of fracture.

6. Wrapping the patient in a blanket can be an effective restraint, and in extreme cases a patient can be pinned in a corner by two or three men holding a mattress.

## WHEN TO USE TRANQUILLISERS

Many patients will calm down with this approach, and in these cases pharmacological management should be avoided. If restraint with medication is required, then it is necessary to make a clinical assessment of the presumed cause of the disturbance.

1. For very anxious or distressed patients a single dose of a benzodiazepine will calm them without altering important diagnostic symptoms or signs. Responding with early medication in this way may help to gain the patient's cooperation with further interviewing and investigation.
2. Where possible neuroleptic drugs should not be given until enough information is available to make a firm diagnosis, and ideally should only be instituted by whoever is responsible for following up the patient.
3. Sedating neuroleptics may exacerbate medical illnesses or produce acute toxic effects.
4. Agitated, or severely disturbed patients will require admission to a psychiatric ward and there is little purpose in giving large doses of neuroleptics before admission.

Management of disturbed patients in whom the diagnosis is clearly established is best done by a combination of containment (observation, limit setting and confinement to a ward if necessary) and fixed, low-dose tranquillisation, using for example chlorpromazine 100 mg 3 to 4 times daily or haloperidol 10 mg 2 to 3 times daily. This can be supplemented with minor tranquillisers in the short term to reduce anxiety and agitation. The practice of 'rapid tranquillisation', giving one or more doses of neuroleptic agent every 30–60 minutes until the patient settles, has no proven therapeutic advantage and more risk of side-effects and may disguise symptoms of delirium or toxic psychoses (q.v.).

The acutely psychotic patient may well require high doses of a major tranquilliser. It is better if a disturbed patient can be persuaded to take oral medication as this implies active cooperation on his part. In this case syrup is preferable as it is easier to be certain that the drug is actually taken. Chlorpromazine 100–200 mg or haloperidol 10–20 mg are effective and relatively safe drugs. The main risk of high doses of chlorpromazine is postural hypotension, and of haloperidol an acute dystonic reaction. This latter can be treated with procyclidine 10 mg given intravenously.

When the patient is struggling, or will not take oral medicines, then the intramuscular route is to be preferred. Haloperidol is a suitable agent and can be given in doses of 5–10 mg. If the patient has known hypersensitivity to major tranquillisers then sodium amytal (up to 500 mg) or valium (10–20 mg) can be used.

The most rapidly effective route for administering drugs is into a vein, using a butterfly cannula rather than a needle attached directly to a syringe, but this can be both difficult and dangerous in a struggling or uncooperative patient.

As well as the side-effects outlined above, sedatives such as benzodiazepines or barbiturates, especially in patients who have been taking other drugs, can cause apnoea requiring assisted ventilation.

## FURTHER TREATMENT

1. Although it is appropriate to deal with legitimate grievances, ward policy or agreed management should never be changed in response to threat.
2. Any patient who has been sedated pharmacologically must be observed closely and their blood pressure,

pulse, respiration and level of consciousness monitored. The patient must be kept in a place where emergency equipment and drugs are readily available so that any adverse effects can be dealt with speedily.

3. Full medical and neurological assessment will need to be carried out and appropriate treatment instituted. When disturbed patients have serious physical illnesses close liaison between medical and psychiatric services may be required.

4. Alternatives to hospital admission should be considered. Resources and support available should be carefully assessed. Telephone numbers of emergency services, including police, social services and Samaritans, should be available in all units.

5. If a secure ward is available with high staffing levels and facilities for careful observation then nursing the patient in such an environment is preferable to relying on high doses of medication or physical restraint.

It may well be that even when admission is considered necessary (or a confused or suicidal patient wants to leave hospital) the patient will not agree to remain in hospital. In this eventuality the patient can be compelled to remain on an involuntary basis under the powers of the Mental Health Act (q.v.). However, informing the patient that you have a legal duty to detain him to prevent him harming himself or others may be sufficient to persuade him to remain without ultimately resorting to the law, but this may raise ethical issues; *see* Chapter 20.

The decision not to admit a potentially violent patient, or the decision to admit someone against their will, both involve a judgement as to the degree of risk of serious violence. The question of involuntary hospitalisation is particularly difficult when the decision has to be based on the presumed risk to others. Some of the factors involved in making such judgements have been outlined above, but ultimately there is no reliable method of assessing dangerousness in any individual. This is a fact of life that has to be tolerated by those involved in making such decisions, but anxiety can be minimised by erring on the side of caution, and perhaps being rather too ready to admit patients, at least in the short term.

## POSTSCRIPT

When a potentially violent incident is over it is important that staff members involved have a few minutes to discuss the incident, both to allow remaining hostile or anxious feelings to be aired and to make the most of the opportunity for learning how to handle any future incidents. Other patients may need to be reassured or given an opportunity to ventilate anxiety or anger.

All incidents involving violence should be carefully recorded as soon as possible after the incident, and reported to others such as unit administrators who may be involved in any sequelae. Any injury to staff should be reported through usual channels. Always remember that incidents involving violence may have legal consequences, not least because individuals involved in such incidents can be litiginous.

# 11. Acute severe stress—victims of abuse and violence

Events which place sudden severe stress on a person's psychological and social functioning include accidents, bereavement, rape and physical abuse. Bereavement and loss are dealt with in a separate chapter; in this chapter some general features of responses to acute stress are outlined, and the problems of rape and physical abuse within families are covered in more detail.

It has become usual practice to distinguish *adjustment disorders* in which patients show unusual (for them) emotional or behavioural responses to stressors from the more severe *post-traumatic stress disorder*. The former are by definition transient and normal functioning returns when the stressor is removed. The appropriate response is crisis intervention (q.v.). More severe stresses can produce enduring symptoms and sometimes gross impairment of normal functioning. DSM-III defines post traumatic stress disorder and offers the following criteria for diagnosis:

1. A recognisable stressor (includes rape, assault, disasters, etc.).
2. Evidence that the patient is re-experiencing the trauma, with recurrent intrusive recollections or recurrent dreams, or is suddenly acting or feeling as if the trauma were reoccurring.
3. The patient has a numbing of responsiveness or reduced involvement with the external world (constricted range of mood, feeling detached or estranged, reduced interest in former activities).

4. At least two of the following are present: hyperalertness or increased startle response; sleep disturbance; guilt about surviving; impaired memory or trouble concentrating; avoiding activities that recall the trauma; intensified symptoms when exposed to events that symbolise or resemble the trauma (e.g. anniversaries, returning to site of assault, physical examination after rape).

There are thus profound effects on the mood, perceptions and behaviour of victims of stressful or violent events. These effects may be seen acutely or may develop over weeks or even months.

a. The victim's *mood* may encompass severe feelings of depression and intense inner pain. There is characteristically a period of numbness and shock. Victims may be frightened or bewildered. There may be rage and indignation, often directed in an ill-focussed way to others around. Most victims feel profoundly helpless in the face of circumstances.

b. The victim's *perceptions* of themselves or others may be altered. They may feel guilty about their imagined contribution to the assault (battered wives believing they 'asked for it'; rape victims castigating themselves for accepting a lift home or an extra drink). There may be profound distrust of others (rape victims can be suspicious of all men, abused children settle into postures of 'frozen watchfulness'). There may be continual reviewing of the event in mental pictures, dreams or nightmares.

c. *Behaviour* can alter in many ways. Normal work or daily routine may not be resumed for some time. Some victims withdraw from others and spend time alone, others desperately seek out the company of others. There may be loss of appetite and sleep disturbance.

These responses will be affected by the victim's basic stance in life (optimistic, pessimistic, religious, etc.) and the strength of their self-image. The relationship to the assailant (relative, friend, boss, etc.), or to significant others (a rape victim may not only feel disgusted with herself but believe that her husband will feel the same way for example) may be important. If the victim is suffering physical pain, emotional reactions will be intensified. Victims may resort to drugs or alcohol to help cope with acute or enduring symptoms following trauma.

Violence and its consequences are not always easy to recognise. Victims may hesitate to report abuse for fear of being blamed, disbelieved or increasing the risk of future violence. Unexplained or unusual injuries or stories that do not fit with the injuries should always be responded to with tactful enquiry about causes.

## RAPE AND SEXUAL ASSAULT

Rape is not just a sexual act but is primarily a crime of violence, an assault on the victim's body and sometimes life. It is a common and much under-reported crime. In the majority of cases force is used, the victim is frequently threatened with a weapon and may be beaten, often severely. The assailant may be a relative or acquaintance, or a total stranger. Victims can be any age, from children to the elderly.

In addition to the general features of post-traumatic stress reaction outlined above, victims of rape understandably have decreased sexual desire or activity with distrust of men. They may have a variety of somatic complaints. Many victims have violent thoughts and wishes, either of revenge or suicide. Recurrent nightmares of the assault are common, and the victim may avoid the scene of the attack, or anything that reminds her of it.

After a period of perhaps several weeks of emotional confusion and disorganisation the 'reorganisation phase' begins. Symptoms will gradually diminish with return to normal functioning, but full recovery can take many months or even years. If the assailant has robbed her, taking for example a handbag with keys and personal information, it may be necessary for the victim to change her door locks or telephone number. Victims often change their lives completely, moving to a new area or changing job.

## APPROACHING THE RAPE VICTIM

The victim must be treated with patience and consideration. Many victims will find it hard to give details of what they have experienced. Quiet, comfort, acceptance and reassurance are essential. The victim's fears and insecurity should be recognised with questions such as 'Do you feel able to talk now?' or 'Do you feel safe now?'. Victims may be angry with staff, or apparently excessively calm. Both these responses should be understood as reactions to stress.

The purpose of the interview should be explained along with the need to ask specific questions, both for the sake of the victim's own health and because of possible legal consequences.

The history should be recorded as far as possible in the victim's own words, and all findings and investigations carefully documented—the notes may be subpoenaed in court. Using the term 'alleged', especially about the assailant prevents prejudice and errs on the side of safety.

Physical examination will be necessary to detect injury and to document evidence of the assault. The victim may feel that physical examination is akin to another rape and must be given sufficient time and information to give proper consent.

The victim must also be given adequate time to make her own decision about whether to involve the police. Until such decision is reached, appropriate samples and all clothing should be kept for possible forensic examination.

If the interviewer is aware of his own possible reactions of anger at the rapist or the victim, embarrassment or prurient interest he will be able to protect the victim from them. Victims are often met with preconceptions amounting to myths about rape, and such responses in staff will greatly hinder effective help being given and should be avoided. It is untrue that all women secretly want to be raped; that women provoke or ask to be raped; that women cannot be raped against their will; or that women passively accept rape. Not all alleged rape actually occurs, but it is very rare for such cases to present to medical services in the first instance.

## MANAGEMENT

Some victims may be reassured by the prescription of medication to prevent pregnancy—the 'morning after pill'. Appropriate physical treatment will be necessary for injuries sustained in the assault.

The meaning of the assault for the victim should be explored, for example feelings of guilt or responsibility can be ventilated. Some women will have a negative self-image of helplessness, weakness or vulnerability reinforced. Some women are most disturbed by the violence of the attack and this must not be underestimated in the exploration of the sexual side.

Crisis intervention techniques (q.v.) of helping the victim identify areas of difficulty and find her own solutions can be useful. Further contacts should be offered, and arranged for any victim who requests it. Anyone who may encounter rape victims should have the telephone number of a rape counselling centre available and offer it to the victim.

Telling the victim what symptoms and personal experiences she might expect, both immediately and in the future, may reassure her and help her feel more in control of her self and her life.

## VIOLENCE WITHIN FAMILIES

The family is the single most frequent site of violence, which may include physical abuse of wives, children, parents or elderly relatives.

Domestic assault is rarely complained of directly. Victims often try to protect the abuser. Presentation may be with depression, somatic complaints, repeat visits with poor compliance with treatment or trivial illnesses in children. Evidence of injury with unconvincing explanations ('I walked into a door'), or injuries at different stages of healing should raise suspicions, as should repeated injuries and repeated presentations, especially with a vague or inconsistent history.

## 'BATTERED WIVES'

Physical abuse of women by their regular partners is common (some 3% of contacts with the Samaritans are for battering). Injuries vary from bruising (in virtually all cases) to fractures, unconsciousness and death. Injuries are most often inflicted to the face or breasts, and often to the abdomen if the victim is pregnant.

Nearly all assaults occur in the house, and it is rare for domestic violence to result in prosecution. Many cases are associated with alcohol consumption by assailant, victim or both. There is a vicious cycle of drinking, mounting tension and relief in violence. Alcohol acts as a disinhibiting agent and also as a convenient excuse for both partners ('He's perfectly alright when he's not drunk').

When violence occurs, it is important to consider both partners and their circumstances. Assault often represents long-standing tensions within the relationship. Both assailant and victim may come from deprived backgrounds where alcohol abuse and violence were prominent.

## CHARACTERISTICS OF THE ASSAILANT

1. History of violence and trouble with the law.
2. Violence is a response to a threat to low self-esteem.
3. Excessively jealous or protective.
4. Usually remorseful and caring after the assault.

## CHARACTERISTICS OF THE VICTIM

1. Often physically or sexually abused in childhood.
2. Low self-esteem and dependency may be prominent.
3. Often rationalises or excuses violence ('It's only when he drinks'; 'He's under a lot of stress').
4. Unreasonable expectations are common ('He's promised not to do it again').

## ASSESSMENT

It is important to avoid the two opposing attitudes (1) that the victim deserves or asks for the assault and (2) that the victim has absolutely no responsibility for the situation. The first is untrue and the second may block off useful avenues for helping the victim understand and gain control of factors in the relationship that lead to violence. If the interviewer is overtly critical of the spouse the victim may begin to defend him.

Presenting complaints may be of marital problems, anxiety or depression. The victim will be anxious and aroused, and may complain of insomnia or nightmares. Abuse of hypnotics, sedatives or analgesics is common. Many victims will be depressed and the risk of suicide should be assessed in all cases (q.v.).

The wife may be frightened to talk about violence for fear of further violence in retaliation. It is necessary to see a woman who is suspected of being a victim alone, and tactful but direct questions should be asked about abuse, including any past injuries, alcohol use and whether anyone else is involved (for example, children).

Domestic violence can escalate and lead to murder. A history of increasing violence, especially involving alcohol and/or weapons should be considered particularly ominous.

If battering occurs for the first time after many years of apparently successful marriage the husband should be investigated for physical or psychiatric illness, head injury or alcoholism.

## TREATMENT

The first need is to treat the physical consequences of the assault. If there is continuing risk, the safety of the wife and children must be ensured.

A factor that correlates with the wife being able to leave the relationship is intervention by helping agencies, but such intervention must be directed towards helping the woman regain control over her own life. Exploring her options, both of staying and leaving, and allowing her to generate possible solutions is the best course. Practical help and advice may have to be given and the emergency telephone numbers of social services and shelters for abused women should be readily available.

Drugs are rarely indicated in the crisis situation, and may be used impulsively for self-harm or suicide.


## CHILD ABUSE

Child abuse, including physical injury, sexual abuse, poisoning or neglect, is a common problem. There are over 3,000 reported cases of severe physical abuse per year in Britain and this probably represents an underestimate of the real incidence.

### PHYSICAL ABUSE

As well as features such as injuries inconsistent with the history and injuries in varying stages of healing there may be delay in seeking medical care. The mother may be distant or tense, with little sign of interaction with or affection towards the child.

ASSESSMENT

The interviewer should remain non-judgemental and aim at building a positive relationship with the parents before confronting them directly with any suspicions. An attitude of inquisition or blame may cause parents to become angry and defensive, denying any harm to the child. Instead the interviewer must try to make sense of the family's difficulties. Children who are provocative, argumentative, subject to temper tantrums or fighting are especially problematic, provoking excessive response from parents. The emphasis should be on trying to help the family with their problem.

Thorough physical examination is essential, including X-rays of limbs and skull, and photographs taken of visible signs of trauma.

TREATMENT

Any acute medical problems must be dealt with, and hospital admission is justified both if it is indicated medically or if there is fear for the child's safety.

Further management should be by the paediatric services, who are experienced with such problems and aware of the complex social and legal procedures that may be involved.

*SEXUAL ABUSE*

Sexual abuse comprises about one-fifth of known cases of child abuse, but is almost certainly under-reported. It may involve masturbation, oral sex or intercourse. Physical complications include venereal disease and pregnancy. Sexual abuse is usually by a close relative or family friend. Incest most commonly involves the father and eldest daughter.

Children rarely report sexual abuse, and false accusations of sexual abuse are rare. However, parents may express disbelief or attempt to discredit the child in an attempt to save their marriage or avoid prosecution. The report of abuse may be a response to the emergence of another family crisis.

There is usually a history of marital or sexual problems, frequently the father complaining of his wife's coldness or distance. The mother often knows about and may collude with incest, but may deny it when asked.

Gynaecological symptoms in a prepubertal child should raise suspicions of sexual abuse. Unexplained changes in behaviour or school performance, and suicidal behaviour are common accompaniments.

ASSESSMENT AND TREATMENT

The approach to the family is similar to that outlined above for physical abuse. Physical examination will be focussed on gynaecological examination and special tests for venereal disease or pregnancy if there is a risk, rather than trauma.

It must be remembered that there is a risk of suicide in all family members after disclosure and appropriate assessment should be made (q.v.). Hospitalisation or fostering of the child might be necessary, or gaining agreement from the family that the father temporarily leaves home.

Referral to paediatric services should be a matter of urgency.

## ABUSE OF THE ELDERLY

There is increasing evidence of abuse, including violence, threats, restraint and negligence, but the overall scale of the problem is unclear. Much of the abuse is overlooked by professionals and concealed by caretakers. The dependency and helplessness of many elderly people, and the apparent hopelessness of the situation, can produce despair, depression and anger in the caretakers. The elderly often have limited contacts outside the home, are ignorant of their legal rights and may be apathetic and debilitated, so their complaints go unheard.

Physical abuse includes burning, beating, scalding, neglect, poor diet and hygiene, and bed sores. Theft, fraud and embezzlement are also common.

## ASSESSMENT

A history should be taken from the patient—it is too easy to get a story from the person escorting the patient and fail to record the specific circumstances of any injury.

Physical examination may reveal bruises, bite marks, burns, lacerations and abrasions, possibly infected. There may be signs of confinement to a chair or bed, or prolonged sitting on the toilet, including sores. There may be other evidence of poor care, including unchanged dressings, dirty or urine-soaked clothing and infected wounds.

The patient may appear nervous and watchful, or fearful of those accompanying him. Fear can be mistaken for paranoid or senile behaviour and ignored.

Other informants, especially caretakers, may seem disinterested or withdrawn, or be aggressive and threatening with the patient.

## TREATMENT

In general it is sufficient for the emergency assessment to recognise the abuse and engage the family in further treatment. Referral to the specialist services for the elderly who are aware of community resources and the need to support caregivers is essential.

# 12. Homelessness and loneliness

There is no clear diagnostic group of patients who present as homeless or isolated, nor is it always the patient himself who initiates the presentation, but other caretakers (family, friends, landlords, wardens). Some of the more common problems that present in this way include:

1. Elderly patients, often with chronic physical illnesses or dementia.
2. Vagrants, often chronically alcoholic or aloof, eccentric and non-comformist.
3. Patients who abuse alcohol and drugs (q.v.), who may present as intoxicated or in acute withdrawal.
4. Patients with abnormal personality (q.v.), often following rejection by others.

## REASONS FOR PRESENTATION

Many of these patients present to medical or other agencies rather than social services because they perceive their problems as illness, or because they lack the knowledge or skill to obtain more appropriate help and the casualty department is immediately accessible. Patients with nowhere to go pose difficulties for a number of reasons:

1. The presentation is usually with symptoms (such as acute anxiety, or exacerbation of long-standing psychiatric illness) that represent the underlying psychosocial crisis rather than a medical or psychiatric emergency.
2. The underlying problems of homelessness or social isolation are frustrating because they are perceived both as serious and threatening difficulties requiring a

response and as irrelevant to emergency medical intervention.

3. Homelessness or loneliness may seem to be the fault of the patient or those close to him, and the apparent attempt to transfer responsibility to helping agencies generates anger and intolerance.

4. There may be a long history of similar presentations where the patient has refused to accept effective help beyond immediate care, and only seeks help when there is a crisis. Chronic alcoholics, vagrants and the chronic mentally ill may adopt this pattern of relating to medical services.

5. There may be reasons why the situation realistically seems hopeless. Patients may anticipate failure, lack both the initiative and the skills to alter their situation. Mental illness, drug or alcohol abuse or a prison record make finding employment, accommodation and friends even less likely.

Patients present as emergencies either in a psychological or social crisis, or suffering from a physical or psychiatric illness. Crises may be associated with any of the following.

## 1. LOSS

a. *Loss of important supportive relationships,* for example following bereavement, separation or divorce. Caretakers may themselves fall ill, or have too many other demands on their resources.

*Case example:* A young woman with a history of multiple overdoses presented having cut her wrists superficially. She was brought by two flatmates who insisted they could no longer 'take responsibility' for her suicidal feelings and did not want her to stay in their flat.

b. *Loss of shelter* following eviction, ejection by relatives, discharge from hospital or prison, or simply moving to a new town.

*Case example:* A 73-year-old woman was brought to casualty by her daughter, having recently been discharged from a hospital in another part of the country. The daughter was angry with the discharge and insistent that she be admitted immediately. On examination the patient had a severe dementia, with no evidence of an acute change in mental functioning. Her 'paranoid' querulousness and suspiciousness was entirely consistent with a long-standing dementing process.

    c. *Loss of personal resources.* This may be due to chronic illness, for example alcoholism or senile dementia, or occur more acutely.

*Case example:* A 45-year-old man left a hostel for alcoholics on a cold January day, caught a train to another city and presented at casualty having spent all his money on drink.

## 2. DESPERATION

    a. Feelings of hopelessness and emptiness, often reinforced by many years of isolation and rejection, can lead to acts of deliberate self-harm. Any homeless or lonely patient should be assessed for risk of suicide (q.v.).
    b. A combination of small events can prove overwhelming, particularly to patients who have spent many years being cared for by others, perhaps in institutions.

*Case example:* A chronic schizophrenic patient presented to casualty requesting admission after he had spent most of his social security allowance and missed the last bus back to his lodging house.

## 3. ILLNESS

Intercurrent physical or psychiatric illnesses can provoke crises in patients otherwise only barely coping.

## 4. THE NEEDS OF OTHERS

Often patients are brought to hospitals or other agencies because those caring for them feel overwhelmed, unsupported or overstretched. The responses of friends or relatives can vary from anger, blame and rejection to involved concern. Some may be totally indifferent and avoid the patient completely. All these responses represent feelings that the demands of the patient outstrip the resources available to meet them.

## ASSESSMENT

As with any patient presenting as an emergency a full assessment is mandatory, including taking a complete history and conducting a physical examination. There is a temptation to be cavalier, offhand or patronising with chronically ill or socially disabled patients. Such a response is degrading and humiliating and must be avoided.

The patient or those accompanying him may present the problem directly ('I've been thrown out of my flat, I need help'), but more usually physical or psychological symptoms will be used as the 'ticket of admission'. Clues may be provided by the manner in which symptoms are presented, for example the patient begins by saying 'I can't cope on my own' or 'I need to be in hospital'. Relatives might begin 'We can't cope with it any more' or 'He can't stay at home, it's making me ill'. The emphasis is on the need for the burden of care to be transferred, rather than on symptoms.

Complaints are often of worsening behaviour such as aggressiveness or wandering at night. The history may give no good evidence of change and there is often an indication of the caretaker having additional needs or problems.

*Case example:* A family brought their elderly mother to hospital requesting admission for 'disturbed' behaviour. It transpired that they were due to go on holiday and the alternative arrangements had broken down at the last minute.

The history should be directed particularly towards eliciting the immediate cause of the crisis including recent events and current supports. Where has the patient been staying and with whom? What resources are available? What other agencies (alcohol treatment units, hospitals, social services, etc.) are involved? How have previous crises been resolved and what are the patient's expectations this time?

Alcohol and substance use, psychiatric and medical history, current mood, any history of self-harm and present suicidal ideas or intentions should be determined. Life-long patterns of vagrancy, loneliness or isolation may be elicited.

The patient's judgement must be evaluated and assessment made of how he is currently handling the crisis. Mental state abnormalities that may interfere with coping, such as hallucinations, disorientation or deficits in cognitive functioning must be determined.

Patients may be angry, hurt or bitter about their experience of loss or rejection. They may feel betrayed by family or friends. They may feel depressed or despairing about their situation. In vagrants or the chronically ill repeated experiences of rejection, homelessness or loss may induce a sense of indifference and apathy. Frequently there are feelings of hopelessness, helplessness and inability to do anything constructive to change their current circumstances. Symptoms of depression should be taken seriously, as a depressive illness might be the reason why the normally tenuous coping has broken down. Suicidal ideation should be responded to as suicide is a real risk.

## MANAGEMENT

### 1. ACUTE MANAGEMENT

The first priority is to provide appropriate treatment for any urgent physical or psychiatric illness. In many cases underlying long-standing difficulties are not susceptible to acute intervention and treatment must focus on the resolution of the current problems, applying the techniques of crisis intervention (q.v.).

In general the problem of homelessness can be met by admission to hospital only if there are appropriate indications (q.v.). Alternatively, after full assessment, the patient can be directed towards other support. All agencies providing an emergency service should have a list of contact telephone numbers for social services, night shelters, nursing homes, helpful landlords and alcohol and drug agencies readily available.

*Loneliness* may not be recognised as a serious difficulty. People who have always had family, friends and a social life may not understand the profound problems these patients have in getting close to others, even to the extent of casual social relationships. Offering simple advice such as 'get out and meet people' or 'join a club' is usually met with apparently insuperable reasons why such suggestions are doomed to failure.

Such attitudes can provoke a 'why bother?' response in those who are being asked to solve the acute problems. Staff soon find themselves in the same position as others who have tried to help—frustrated, angry and rejecting, and ultimately reinforcing the experience of loneliness. In the short term a brief interview with acceptance and understanding of the patient's feelings and the offer of longer-term help is usually sufficient to alleviate the crisis.

## 2. FURTHER CARE

For most patients dealing with the crisis will be all they require or request. Many patients with chronic illnesses will be in current treatment and the appropriate agencies should be informed of the emergency contact and asked to see the patient early if necessary. Any other agency to whom the patient has been directed should be contacted, preferably by telephone to ensure adequate continuity of care.

For lonely, isolated patients the emergency contact may be

a first step in admitting the need for more intensive help. Too rapid an approach may stir up the patient's fears of closeness and may prevent them engaging in treatment. It may be helpful to allow the patient to return a few times to talk about their loneliness to establish the contact before making a referral to local psychiatric or psychotherapy services.

# Part D
# Psychiatric disorders in general medical settings

# 13. Psychiatric disorder presenting with physical symptoms

Very many patients present to medical services with physical symptoms which have no apparent organic basis. These symptoms may be transient or develop into a chronic and incapacitating way of life. Sometimes these patients present as emergencies, but more commonly the 'emergency' arises when investigations fail to uncover an obvious cause for the complaints. The patient's insistent demands for relief of symptoms coupled with staff frustration at the apparent impossibility of providing such relief often leads to the request for urgent psychiatric intervention. This is only too often a routine request to the duty psychiatrist, himself often busy and relatively inexperienced, who responds by excluding affective disorders and psychosis and leaves the (frustrating and irritating) comment 'No formal psychiatric illness' recorded in the medical notes.

This stage, at which physical investigations are completed, is crucial in the treatment of patients who present psychological problems as somatic distress. Accepting this and responding with patience and sympathetic attempts to understand why this patient is presenting in this way can make the difference between effective treatment and failure with mutal anger and recrimination. Often these problems cannot be assessed fully as an emergency, but require admission for investigation and the initiation of treatment.

It is important to recognise that these patients are suffering from psychiatric illness. Their symptoms are not under voluntary control, nor are they 'imaginary' in the sense that this term is commonly used. It is more useful to accept that all pain and distress is perceived and interpreted through higher centres in the central nervous system, and that pain so perceived is 'real' whatever the cause. There is no difference in the pain felt in the toes of a real limb or an amputated limb. Ultimately 'all pain is psychological'.

## ASSESSMENT

Patients may present somatic symptoms as a representation or screen for a wide variety of psychosocial problems. It is important to assess for possible physical illness, but also to allow sufficient time, and be sufficiently receptive, for the patient to ventilate and discuss any such problems.

### DISTINGUISHING PHYSICAL AND PSYCHIATRIC ILLNESS

Recognition of a psychiatric cause for physical symptoms must follow, not precede, exclusion of organic pathology. The first stage therefore is to decide whether an organic basis for the symptoms can be discovered. It is not uncommon for patients with serious and treatable physical illnesses to be diagnosed as 'hysterical', especially if the symptoms are vague, non-specific or fluctuating in severity (for example multiple sclerosis or myasthenia gravis).

Lack of firm evidence of organic pathology is not a sufficient reason to assume an illness is psychological. There must be adequate reasons for such a decision. Functional illness may be suspected if:

1.  The symptoms are ill-defined and do not correspond to known anatomical or physiological functioning. They may be vague or changeable. Special investigations are characteristically negative.
2.  The severity of the symptoms is inconsistent with the severity of impairment of occupational or social functioning.
3.  There is evidence of psychosocial stress related in time

to the onset of symptoms. Sometimes symptoms vary with the immediate situation.

4. There is evidence of suggestibility. Patients give positive responses to direct questions about symptoms.

5. There may be a 'model' for the symptoms, someone close to the patient who has had similar symptoms in the past. A clear example is the common finding that recently bereaved patients present with physical symptoms similar to those suffered by their relative before death.

6. It may be helpful to find evidence that the symptoms are helping to solve a psychological conflict experienced by the patient, but in practice such 'primary gain' is difficult to elicit in a convincing fashion.

7. The interviewer may get the feeling that the patient is concerned with trying to convince him of the reality of the symptoms. Patients are often very alert to any hint of doubt in the interviewer's tone or manner.

The idea that if symptoms are used to obtain a caring, supportive or emotional response from others (so-called 'secondary gain' or 'attention-seeking') this indicates functional rather than organic illness is a serious mistake. These concepts require a subjective judgement on the part of the assessor as to how appropriate the behaviour is in the circumstances. Patients with acute appendicitis could be said to be seeking attention (in this case from the surgeon) and obtaining secondary gain (care from nurses and family, time off work). This is clearly worlds apart from a patient who is responding to early childhood neglect or deprivation by eliciting care from others and simultaneously expressing hidden anger and resentment by provoking irritation and helpless frustration in staff in the 'parental' or authority role. It is better to understand that all patients are seeking attention and to try and understand what attention they need and why they are seeking it at this time.

There are twin dangers at this stage of assessment. The first is to attribute psychological causes to symptoms as soon as investigations prove negative: diagnosis by exclusion rather than inclusion. The second is to assume that if there are good reasons to diagnose either a physical or a psychiatric cause for the symptoms then the other class of diagnosis is excluded. In fact both can occur together, for example in multiple sclerosis or epilepsy.

Symptoms of physical and psychiatric illnesses can occur in a variety of combinations:

1. Physical illnesses can be exacerbated by psychiatric disturbance.
2. Physical illness can produce secondary psychiatric disturbance.
3. Psychiatric illness may present with somatic symptoms.
4. Unrelated physical and psychiatric disturbances may occur coincidentally.


*THE PSYCHIATRIC DIAGNOSIS*

Various attempts have been made to classify somatic presentations of psychological disorders, and we have adopted the general term 'somatoform disorders' used in the American DSM-III system. This system subclassifies these disorders (*see Table* 13.1), but in practice, especially in the emergency setting, such distinctions are bedevilled by descriptive difficulties and are of little help.

The sociological concepts of the 'sick role' (referring to the situation where a sick person is allowed to shed social, family and occupational responsibilities) and 'abnormal illness behaviour' (where patients cling to the sick role inappropriately) have been useful, but have increasingly come to carry judgemental overtones. There is a tendency to equate the sick role with being inadequate or ineffective, and illness behaviour with malingering. Nonetheless, putting a patient's

*Table* 13.1 SOMATOFORM DISORDERS (BASED ON DSM-III)

1. *Conversion disorder* (monosymptomatic):
Alteration of physical functioning as an expression of psychological need. Commonly involves voluntary motor system and sensory organs. Onset usually sudden. Symptoms frequently suggest neurological disease. Impairment does not conform to recognised anatomical function.

2. *Psychogenic pain disorder* (pain):
Similar to conversion. Pain is the predominant or only symptom.

3. *Somatisation disorder* (Briquet's syndrome) (polysymptomatic):
Chronic, fluctuating course. Onset before 30 years. Almost always women. Many medical evaluations and surgical procedures. Multiple symptoms, including pain in any system, cardiovascular, respiratory or neurological symptoms and psychosexual dysfunction.

4. *Hypochondriasis*:
Patients believe they have serious physical disease, become preoccupied with health, misinterpret minor signs and symptoms and cannot be reassured.

5. *Factitious disorders*:
Repeated presentation with physical symptoms (Munchausen's syndrome) or psychological symptoms (Ganser's syndrome). Symptoms under voluntary control. The reasons for the conscious simulation are not immediately apparent. Patients seem to crave admission.

6. *Malingering*:
Presentation with physical symptoms under conscious control. The gain is usually obvious to the observer. The patient is reluctant to accept extensive or painful procedures (unlike factitious disorders).

symptoms and his responses to them into a social context is an important part of assessment and treatment.

The differential diagnosis of somatoform disorder includes a number of psychiatric illnesses which may present with somatic complaints. These include:

1. *Schizophrenia.* There may be multiple somatic complaints, often bizarre.
2. *Monosymptomatic delusional states.* There is a single symptom, held with delusional intensity. May be bizarre.

3. *Depression.* Somatic symptoms may be an expression of distress, or part of the illness, such as the nihilistic delusions in depressive psychosis ('My insides have rotted away', 'I'm going to die'). Commonly, depressive illnesses exacerbate the symptoms of, or reduce the patient's ability to cope with, a coexisting physical illness.

4. *Anxiety.* Symptoms are usually related to autonomic arousal (*see* Chapter 6). Phobias about cancer or other illnesses have a similar form to other phobias (q.v.).

5. *Alcohol abuse* can present both with physical symptoms in the absence of organic pathology and as physical illnesses secondary to alcohol abuse.

6. Patients in *psychosocial crisis* may present with somatic symptoms.

## TREATMENT

In the emergency setting, or wherever an urgent response is expected, patients presenting with somatic symptoms can prove both difficult and frustrating for staff. They have enduring complaints, sometimes serious (blindness, severe weight loss) but often seemingly 'exaggerated' responses to relatively 'trivial' pathology (severe abdominal pain with no demonstrable organic basis). When no organic cause is found staff may feel they are being deceived and become angry, offering inadequate assessment and early discharge. On the other hand, some patients find a doctor who rises to the clinical challenge and pursues a prolonged, elaborate but fruitless programme of investigation and treatment.

The stage when physical investigations are complete is crucial in management of these patients. It is at this point that (a) staff feel sufficiently confident that serious organic pathology is excluded and (b) patients can be offered an alternative model of illness and treatment that might prove beneficial. Spending a little extra time at this stage can avoid premature termination of treatment. There are two stages to this approach:

1. *The reality of the patient's symptoms and suffering must be openly acknowledged.* Patients are very sensitive to any suggestion that 'It's all in the mind' or 'There's nothing really wrong'. However, it is also important to avoid colluding with patients by agreeing with their understanding of the origin of the symptoms. The best attitude is one of 'puzzled concern' ('Well you'll be pleased to hear that the tests we've done don't show any really serious problems such as cancer. We need to talk a bit more about where we go from here'). Facing the patient directly with the absence of organic pathology and the need to obtain a psychiatric opinion usually leads to the patient leaving treatment and trying to find a more sympathetic doctor.

2. *Psychological and physical factors contributing to symptoms need to be related to each other in a way the patient can understand.* This topic can be introduced in terms of the doctor's interest in the relationship between mind and body, using common examples, for instance tension headaches, or low mood and lethargy following influenza. Often the patient will be able to relate changes in symptoms to other factors ('I do get indigestion when I'm under stress at work': 'It has been much worse since I've been worried about my daughter'). Thus the diagnosis is 'reframed' in terms which consider the patient as a whole and do not dismiss psychological factors as 'all in the mind' and therefore irrelevant.

Definitive treatment can rarely be offered in an emergency setting. The patient may require prolonged assessment, but even when this is completed in many cases management will require contact with the patient lasting many months or perhaps years. The main function of emergency intervention is to establish the basis for enduring treatment. Useful rules include:

1. Any hint of hostility, disinterest or outright rejection must be avoided.
2. Reassurance that there is 'nothing wrong' and that symptoms will improve may make the interviewer feel better but will be proved wrong more often than not.
3. It is often better to aim for improvement in function rather then relief of symptoms.
4. The temptation to pursue symptomatology with ever more elaborate investigations should be resisted.
5. Medication should be avoided where possible.

A minority of patients will accept the findings of physical investigations and accept that they 'just have to live with' their symptoms. If the acute presentation seems to be related to specific life stresses then crisis intervention techniques (q.v.) can be helpful. If there is evidence of formal psychiatric illness such as depression, anxiety or psychosis then appropriate treatment or referral should be offered (q.v.).

Otherwise the best treatment is usually offered by a sympathetic doctor who is able to follow up the patient for a long time, maintaining an attitude of therapeutic optimism without giving up hope when physical symptoms do not improve. Such treatment will allow the patient to review his symptoms, but aim primarily at improvement in function. The person in the best position to offer such follow-up is the patient's general practitioner.

Direct referral to a psychiatrist is often resisted, and may damage the relationship between patient and doctor ('He just thinks I'm crazy'). There is often too great an expectation of psychiatrists in these cases, a feeling that once the 'psychological causes' have been discovered by experts then the patient will be cured. In fact only too often the psychiatrist can offer little more then the exclusion of psychiatric diagnoses such as depression. Insight orientated psychotherapy is generally of little help, and general practitioners can offer better continuity of care.

The main complications of treatment are iatrogenic. Dependence on analgesics or minor tranquillisers can readily develop. Some patients undergo repeated invasive investigations or even surgical procedures.

## FACTITIOUS DISORDERS AND MALINGERING

These conditions are relatively uncommon but are important to recognise. In both cases symptoms are under voluntary control, but patients with factitious disorders ('Munchausen's syndrome') have no immediately apparent reason for simulating symptoms. Malingerers feign illness for gain and in many cases this is obvious to observers.

### *MUNCHAUSEN'S SYNDROME*

This is a disorder that is puzzling and frustrating to treat, and often leads to rejection of the patient. These patients gain repeated admission for physical symptoms, usually those of severe illnesses. There is no obvious gain from the symptoms, but a craving for admission. Patients willingly undergo painful or dangerous procedures (for instance laparotomy, craniotomy or tracheostomy). They often have an abdomen criscrossed with scars.

Although their symptoms are seen to be under voluntary control this is usually only an inference by an outside observer. There may be an analogy with compulsive behaviour (q.v.) which is experienced by the patient as voluntary action, but irresistable and therefore beyond control.

The main areas of complaint include:

1. *Abdominal pain,* often mimicking intestinal obstruction or renal colic.
2. *Haemorrhages,* often following self-inflicted wounds in orifices, or blood in urine.
3. *Neurological* —headaches, seizures, sensory loss.
4. *Cardiovascular or respiratory,* for example convincing simulations of myocardial infarction or pulmonary embolus.
5. *Skin lesions,* which may be self-induced by injection, scratching or burning.
6. *Infection*—self-injection can give fevers or abscesses.
7. *Medication abuse,* for example anticoagulant abuse presenting as bleeding disorder.

These patients travel widely and have been admitted to many different hospitals. They may be vague or non-specific about their past medical history, or give a convincing but unverifiable account (for example, records lost in fires or recent arrival from another country). They often show great familiarity with medical terms and procedures. They may lie in a dramatic and extremely convincing manner. They often have a background in work in a medical field or hospital related activity. There may be a history of drug abuse (often analgesics).

If admitted these patients usually become increasingly hostile, belligerent and demanding, provoking an extreme negative response from staff. They frequently take their own discharge, especially when confronted with the suspicion that their symptoms are feigned.

There may be evidence from the history or the patient's behaviour of three possible psychological motivations. Being cared for often seems to provide intense gratification. This may be combined with an apparent wish to be punished by undergoing painful procedures, and a need to frustrate and anger those in authority. All of these could stem from isolation, deprivation or neglect in early childhood.

## MALINGERING

Malingering is a common problem in emergency medicine. There is usually evidence of apparent gain from the symptoms, and patients are reluctant to accept extensive or painful procedures.

The diagnosis can only be confirmed by the patient's confession, which is rarely obtained—confrontation is more likely to lead to the patient storming out, putting all the blame on the staff.

Factitious disorders and malingering do not respond well to medical intervention. This is because the behaviour is a problem for the staff, not the patient, for whom it is a means to an end. Treatment should be aimed at establishing a stable relationship with the patient, avoiding consultation with other agencies, further investigation and treatment as far as possible. Where there is clear evidence of gain (for example a claim for compensation) this should be resolved wherever possible, although this by no means always leads to resolution of symptoms.

# 14. Disturbed patients on medical wards

Any psychiatric syndrome can occur coincidentally with illness requiring in-patient medical treatment, or psychiatric disorder may arise from medical treatment or from other illness-related factors. Investigations, operative procedures or acute medical conditions can be stressful and there are varying degrees of personal vulnerability to these. Good practice requires sufficient sensitivity in staff to detect understandable anxieties and to provide appropriate information about diagnosis and treatment (*see* Chapter 21).

The ability of staff to deal with, and their tolerance towards, symptoms of anxiety and depression varies greatly; where disturbed behaviour (wandering, agitation, threats of suicide, interference with other patients, aggression) is present few wards dealing with the acutely ill can spare staff to deal with prolonged disturbance.

Disturbed patients often invoke a 'telegraphic' style of communication to psychiatrists from acute surgical or medical wards ('He's refusing to stay, and threatening to overdose again. . . Should he be sectioned?'). This commonly may reflect:

a. direct concern for the safety of the patient;
b. anxiety about being responsible if the patient or others come to harm;
c. feelings of inadequacy or helplessness arising from an inability to persuade the patient to stay—this may generate anxiety or a degree of resentment or anger which can lead to:
d. punitive (hostile and rejecting) feelings. The patient should as a matter of course be protected from these as

148

they are rarely constructive (therapeutic)—it may help to divert or reflect these feelings back to the patient in a useful way (*see* Chapter 3);

   e. a lack of confidence (or a reasonable fear of injury) over how much physical restraint may be used;

   f. a tendency to accept greater responsibility for the patient's actions than is reasonably justified;

   g. an intolerance of emotional problems or of patients not showing the expected deference to staff.

There are other possibilities. A request for psychiatric help on general medical and surgical wards does not imply that any of the above is true in the particular case for which help is sought. The degree of urgency should be assesssed in the standard way by obtaining details of the history of the problem; the duty psychiatrist should always speak to the doctor immediately responsible for the patient. If a psychiatric opinion cannot be obtained at once then telephone advice about immediate management should be requested. It is unsatisfactory for a senior house officer in psychiatry, who may have only a few months more experience than the responsible house officer, to provide such guidance unless this is immediately covered by advice from a career registrar or the consultant.

It has to be recognised that one common reason for referral is to obtain the removal of a disruptive patient from the general to a psychiatric ward, and that staff on the general ward may not be receptive to suggestions as to how they should manage the patient. Not infrequently psychiatric help is sought late when the tolerance of the staff has been exhausted, and it is important that the psychiatrist responds in a constructive rather than a critical way to the difficulties.

The evaluation of the patient is essentially the same as that described in the early chapters of this book. The following points can be made:

1. Time should be taken to review the notes and drug charts. Trends may be detected from comments on the behaviour of the patient, his physical status, and the treatment.

2. Medical or surgical treatment may not always be faultless. The psychiatrist and the medical house officer or registrar should always discuss the case together.

3. The nurse in charge and, if possible, the relatives should always be consulted about recent changes in the patient's mood, behaviour, judgement and orientation, and about practical management difficulties. The general practitioner may have useful knowledge of the patient.

4. Simple causes of disturbance should be sought first—pain on a ward where some discomfort or pain is common, or pain arising from operative complications (haematoma or fistulae from stoma construction; peritoneal irritation from failure of sutures in abdominal operations) can, in error, be classed as 'normal', or be attributed to some personal problem. Probably fewer mistakes are made by believing patients and their relatives than the reverse. Factors arising from admission to hospital, especially withdrawal from alcohol or other drugs, should always be considered; disorientation may indicate an early dementia hardly noticed at home.

5. Psychiatric treatment should not be suggested if it is incompatible with other medical or surgical management.

## REFERRAL TO A PSYCHIATRIST

There are still negative connotations in referral to a psychiatrist, arising from the association with 'mental illness' rather than 'emotional problems'. In practice most patients are willing and often relieved to talk about how they feel and how events in their lives are affecting them.

Some psychiatrists accommodate their colleagues in other disciplines and allow themselves to be presented as 'another specialist', a 'nerve doctor' or just 'a colleague'. This type of deception can hardly ever be justified and is a poor basis for the honest relationship required. Before referring the patient agreement to see a psychiatrist must be obtained. If this is not done the important initial relationship may be less easy to establish or, at worst, the patient may abandon all medical investigation and treatment.

*Case example:* A 26-year-old woman with no previous psychiatric history had extensive investigations for disturbed functions of the bowel and had clearly become upset by what are reasonably regarded as uncomfortable and potentially embarrassing procedures. The findings were negative but the problems persisted; she was referred for psychiatric opinion without explanation or agreement. The psychiatrist did not check beforehand that she had agreed to see him. He was unable to sustain the interview after his identity became clear and she left the hospital.

This experience arising from clumsy management could well have many consequences over the years both in terms of her own health and also in her attitude to seeking medical help for her family. Clearly there will be exceptions—in cases of delirium for example—but there is another good reason for adherence to this principle of 'informed consent' to a psychiatric referral. It is the need to consider the reasons for referral in terms understandable to the patient and to convey these to the patient in an acceptable and positive way. The referring doctor must try to ascertain the reasons for distress and present a reasoned case for referral.

## RECORDING A PSYCHIATRIC OPINION

Brevity (rarely more than one half of an A4 sheet), absence of jargon or psychodynamic speculation and clear suggestions are required. The detail usual in a psychiatric history should be recorded in separate psychiatric notes. If possible ICD-9 or DSM-III diagnostic categories should be used. A statement of the psychiatrist's intentions in terms of review or other arrangements for future involvement must be included. If the patient does not fit into any of the common psychiatric syndromes then an explanation of the disturbed behaviour and suggestions as to management should be offered. 'Not psychiatrically ill' is both annoying and unhelpful to staff trying to deal with behaviour they experience as requiring management outside their professional skills.

# 15. The patient who is dying or seriously ill

The section of this book covering staff responses to emotionally difficult situations (Chapter 3) is relevant when considering the care of the seriously ill or dying, since the attitudes of staff and patient may vary considerably and both may use similar protective mechanisms to deal with uncomfortable feelings. In most instances referral to a psychiatrist will be inappropriate and it should only be when the level of emotional distress or disturbance is not responding to the staff's best efforts at intervention that the question of such referral should be raised with the patient.

Maguire has described how staff cope with their own strong feelings when faced with dying patients by using 'distancing tactics'. These include:

1. *False reassurance*, especially about the effectiveness of treatment for pain or other distressing symptoms ('We'll soon have the vomiting under control').
2. *Selective attention*, for example dealing with physical problems and ignoring the psychological message (Patient: 'I'm sure I'm not going to get better—the pain keeps getting worse.' Doctor: 'Is the pain still in the same place?').
3. *'Jollying along'*—responding inappropriately to emotional cues ('Come on now, there's no need to be such a misery').
4. *Avoiding* dying patients by spending less time with them, putting them in side rooms, allowing the ward round to pass by without stopping.

Staff fear getting too close to dying patients because they feel it might cause the patient to be overcome by distress or despair; or that they would in some way harm the patient; or that they might not be able to cope with their own feelings. This last is especially true if the staff member likes the patient, or is reminded by them of someone they are close to , such as a parent.

Sometimes staff avoid discussion because it faces them with problems with which they feel unable to cope. They may not feel they have the appropriate skills to answer questions such as 'How long have I got?'. They may be constrained by instructions from senior staff or relatives not to tell the patient the truth. Staff in general medicine and surgery may be bound by their particular consultant's attitudes. For example, a junior house officer can be placed in a difficult situation when the patient has been told 'It's just a little fluid in the lung' but during the third pleural aspiration asks the direct question 'Have I got cancer?'.

One problem is that senior staff may have good reasons for their position. For example, a consultant may well have in mind that it is better for a patient with diabetic complications requiring amputation of the leg to come to that conclusion himself. If the consultant does not discuss his rationale with his staff thay may wonder why the patient is not advised to have the limb amputated to save his lingering discomfort and immobility. In general patients will reach their own decisions more rapidly and with less distress if they are offered the opportunity to talk and ask questions. Letting the patient make up his own mind may merely be another distancing tactic.

In the case of the house officer aspirating the chest the best course in the first instance (as questions like this are often unexpected initially) is to say that the consultant in charge prefers details of the diagnosis and treatment to be discussed directly with him. If the consultant does not deal with these problems himself he may have to be approached and the issue raised with him. In many instances, more realistically, the house officer will have to involve the registrar or senior registrar, or even just deflect questions and resolve to practise differently himself. It is never permissible to lie to patients, and if faced with direct questions it is best to be honest.

Surveys have shown that the majority of patients wish to know their diagnosis but that is not a guide to the management of the individual patient. Lack of information and avoiding discussion can be potent sources of distress and the general rule is to enable the patient to absorb details of his condition in small steps at his own pace.

For example, after a biopsy the patient may ask 'Can you tell me the result of the test?' to which the doctor may respond 'Some of the cells are a little abnormal.' The first interview may end at that stage. Alternatively either immediately, or on the next day, the patient may ask for more information: 'What do you mean, abnormal? Is it serious, Doctor?' Note that the patient has not used the word cancer—neither should the doctor in his reply: 'If the number of abnormal cells increases they may cause damage.' Patient: 'It's cancer, isn't it?' Again the patient may clearly indicate a wish to leave it there or pursue the topic further. The doctor should say that he will come again to talk the next day about what should be done, as it is best to give opportunity to talk even if little further information is asked for.

## GENERAL RULES FOR INTERVIEWS WITH DYING PATIENTS OR THEIR RELATIVES

1. Always find a quiet, private place to talk.
2. Give patients or relatives an opportunity to express their own feelings.
3. Give information directly and honestly, but *pause* for a response.
4. Do not offer reassurance unless you are sure you are right—for example, do not promise relief from drug side-effects if this is unlikely.
5. Comment on non-verbal cues about feelings ('It seems you've been very worried about it').

6. Be optimistic but honest about treatment and prognosis, giving any positive factors first. Hope is important in avoiding depression.
7. Do not attempt to offer an exact prognosis. No one can ever predict the future and raising false hopes or expectations will not help. Predictions may be self-fulfilling.
8. Stay with the patient or relative until they indicate they have finished asking questions and have been able to acknowledge and share their feelings.

If the patient who is dying has sufficient information the subject of dying may be raised by the patient. Kubler Ross found the most helpful question was 'Do you want to talk about it?' This opportunity can be a release for the patient but again should be at the patient's instigation and not pressed as a necessary stage to pass through. Discussion of fears such as pain or choking can be helpful if this is mentioned by the patient. It should be borne in mind that relatives may use the same defensive and distancing tactics as staff and may need help with their own distress. Later talk can be directed to positive aspects concerned with living.

Tidying affairs can bring a welcome feeling of control and some positive reflections. It must not be assumed that making a will is necessarily a morbid act. Coping with imminent death is clearly a personal affair and care must be taken not to assume a religious or other stance towards death that might reduce the patient's range of coping strategies.

As well as dealing directly with patient's feelings of misery or hopelessness it is important to recognise that dying patients often become depressed. The symptoms of depressive illness (q.v.) must be recognised and appropriate intervention offered. It is too easy, and very common, for patients to attempt to hide their depression, or for staff to assume the depression is 'understandable' ('I'd be depressed too, if I had cancer') and therefore does not require treatment.

In fact, offering an antidepressant appropriately to such patients not only improves their mood, but makes it easier for them to deal with the many tasks facing a dying person such as saying goodbye to their families. Depression makes it more difficult to cope with symptoms such as pain or distressing drug side-effects, and there is evidence that improving a patient's mood also improves the prognosis.

Finally, always involve the family, who may themselves feel they require support but will benefit most if they can be encouraged in turn to provide most of the support required by the patient. Relatives may have strong feelings about whether to tell the patient the diagnosis, and in general their decision should be respected as they know the patient and may be in the best position to judge his needs.

# Part E
# Patients who harm themselves

# 16. The management of deliberate self-harm

In one year about one in eleven of the population will have experienced thoughts ranging from ideas that life is no longer worthwhile to serious contemplation of suicide (1 in 100). A district general hospital serving a population of 250,000 can anticipate 600 referrals annually of persons who have harmed themselves either by self-poisoning or in some other way, and there will be 15 completed suicides in that district. Each health authority is required to develop a policy for the management of patients who harm themselves which must include 'complete physical and psychosocial assessment, treatment and after-care'.

The early statement of policy that all cases of self-harm should be assessed by a psychiatrist was never fully implemented and it is now accepted in practice, supported by research, that an adequate psychosocial assessment can be made by suitable trained hospital medical staff, nurses, or social workers, with referral to a psychiatrist when appropriate.

## PSYCHOSOCIAL ASSESSMENT

The aims are to:

- a. understand the events leading to the self-harm;
- b. determine the mental state;
- c. identify any psychiatric condition;
- d. obtain background details including past psychiatric history and present social circumstances;
- e. with some knowledge of special risk factors evaluate the likelihood of further self-harm or suicide.

161

The requirements are:

a. time for an unhurried interview;
b. a patient who has overcome any initial distress and who is not drowsy or emotionally labile as a result of intoxication with drugs or alcohol;
c. a degree of privacy and freedom from interruption if relevant personal information is to be disclosed;
d. an independent history from a friend or relative as well as any information the GP can provide.

## THE INTERVIEW

Rapport must be established. It may be more successful to ask the individual about feelings and events in the preceding 24–48 hours rather than asking directly about the incident of self-harm immediately.

*You must have been very upset. . . can you tell me whether you were feeling like this a few days ago or was it just tonight? It would help me to understand what has been happening to you if we started on (say) Tuesday morning. . . . Did you get up as usual, have breakfast. . . . What happened then?*

This approach not only allows the patient to put his action into context but also will provide an indication as to whether the event has been within a period of a sustained low mood (which may indicate severe depression) or was a response to a particular situation (more commonly).

## UNDERSTANDING THE EVENT

A clear description of the behaviour leading to the self-harm should be obtained—minute by minute if necessary—with specific attention to attempts to conceal the act, the writing of a note, or elaborate preparations. It is important to elicit, in similar detail, the events which resulted in the person attending the hospital; whether being found by chance or, more often, because the patient has told a friend or relative about the self-harm.

With care this interview, although thorough, need not appear like an interrogation; from time to time it is useful to recapitulate with the patient and try to ascertain the thoughts and feelings that led to or were associated with specific acts. The interviewer could speculate on how the patient may have felt, but this should be done sparingly, avoiding the temptation to provide explanations.

At this stage the interviewer should have an understanding of the details of the act, including a precipitant, and also of the nature of the intent. There are a number of general reasons people recognise in their own motivation—based on their feelings at the time, and also on the wish to influence others. Talking about these possible reasons can increase the information obtained, and may also stimulate the insight of the patient.

*POINTS*

1. If no understandable precipitant has been elicited then it is necessary to consider that:
   a. a more serious reason is being concealed (perhaps domestic or forensic problems); probing into the social and other background history and an interview with an independent informant are required;
   b. there may be a mental illness present, which should be evident in the mental state examination.

2. Use of alcohol must always be ascertained—both general drinking habits and drinking before the act of self-harm.

*MENTAL STATE EXAMINATION (SEE ALSO CHAPTER 1)*

Information on appearance and general behaviour, talk and mood will already have been ascertained from the interview. Closer attention now needs to be given to present thoughts:

1. Main preoccupations and worries, including thoughts of suicide and intentions. Ask specifically about how the future is seen—does everything seem hopeless?
2. Perception of self both before the act of self-harm and at present. Are there thoughts of being a burden, or of being useless?
3. Abnormal beliefs or experiences—severe depression may be accompanied by paranoid delusions, nihilistic delusions or derogatory auditory hallucinations. Some chronic schizophrenic patients may present after an overdose during a relapse of their illness when hallucinations become intrusive and unbearable. Usually these symtoms will be reported but direct questions will be necessary if the patient is withdrawn and uncommunicative.

## INSIGHT

This is best considered after an evaluation of the risk of further self-harm from the history and examination, and after talking with the patient about his ideas on what is needed to help him and his choice of the options available.

## IDENTIFICATION OF PSYCHIATRIC ILLNESS

Diagnosis in psychiatry, like any other diagnosis in medicine, is dependent upon an adequate hisotry. Depressive symptoms are understandably common in this group of patients, and information from friends or relatives should help in distinguishing between relative transient depressive symptoms arising from a personal crisis and the more sustained disturbance of mood associated with anorexia, weight loss, poor concentration, disturbed sleep and loss of interest, present for days or weeks before the self-harm, indicating a major depressive illness (q.v.). Sometimes, more often in younger patients, symptoms may be atypical with weight gain (eating for 'comfort') and isolation by remaining in bed.

Alcoholism, schizophrenia, epilepsy, and early dementia are also associated with an increased risk of suicide.

Anxiety and depression can be difficult to distinguish and as symptoms can accompany most psychiatric syndromes. Anxiety and restlessness when prominent may arise within one or two days in abstinent patients dependent on alcohol or other drugs (q.v.).

Patients with disorders of personality (q.v.) commonly suffer from depressive symptoms and problems in personal relationships with an increased risk of (usually) impulsive self-harm under stress. Evidence of disturbed behaviour from adolescence is necessary to confirm a diagnosis of disordered personality, which is sometimes made too readily, creating a therapeutic nihilism which may be misplaced.

*BACKGROUND*

1. *Psychiatric history.* Details of any previous hospital admissions for mental disorder or treatment as a psychiatric out-patient or referral to a psychologist. Any involvement with the law.
2. *Family psychiatric history.* Has anyone suffered from alcoholism, depression or died from suicide?
3. *Social circumstances.* Has the patient anywhere to stay on discharge? Particularly, is anyone living with the patient? On discharge will a friend or relative be present to go home with the patient? Are there any immediate problems with children, finances, housing department, social services, neighbours?
4. An individual's own perception of his situation, resources and ability to cope, including how similar problems were dealt with in the past.

*EVALUATION OF THE RISK OF FURTHER SELF-HARM*

Various factors relating to the individual (age, presence of mental disorder, certain character traits) and to the situation (living alone, recently bereaved) are associated statistically with an increased risk of repeating an act of self-harm or committing suicide after an earlier episode of self-harm. Similar behaviour, however, has unique determinants for the individual which are only accessible indirectly from the patient.

It is important to cultivate the skill to pursue vague answers to questions about future suicidal intent in a manner which enables the patient to be frank about how he feels but does not encourage spurious responses—for example, the denial of future plans of self-poisoning. 'It can be difficult to say how you will feel in 2–3 days, but what about now?' 'If you did feel suicidal later would you contact the department or a friend?'

Factors associated with serious suicidal intent and risk of further self-harm are:

1. The event:
   —Evidence of careful planning.
   —Precautions to avoid discovery.
   —Elaborate method (combined overdose and drowning).
   —Use of violence (hanging, jumping from high building, severe cuts, use of fire).
   —No obvious precipitant.
2. Mental state:
   —Retardation or agitation; resentful and uncooperative.
   —Depression with sense of hopelessness and 'black' future; guilt, feeling a burden; anger (particularly in the young); low esteem.
   —Regret at not having been successful (suicide); plans to complete the act (particularly if these ideas persist over several days of admission).
   —Delusions associated with religious ideas; premonition of cataclysmic events (end of world) with thoughts of having failed God; any identification with Satan; ideas related to wickedness, punishment

and sin—sometimes can lead to mutilation of offending part (eye, hand, genitals); delusions associated with depression, e.g. unrealistic assessment of future, nihilistic delusions, having venereal disease.

3. Background:
   —Middle age (over 35).
   —Male sex.
   —Unemployment; loss of job.
   —Living alone; social isolation; little social support.
   —Recent separation or bereavment.
   —History of mental illness (depression; alcoholism).
   —Previous episode of deliberate self-harm.
   —Suicide in first degree relative.
   —Severe (terminal) illness in the elderly.

## PSYCHIATRIC ILLNESS ASSOCIATED WITH SUICIDE

1. *Severe depression.* The intensity of 'mild' depression (dysthymia—q.v.) may briefly exceed that experienced in the more prolonged and sustained major depressive illnesses (q.v.), which respond to antidepressant medication and ECT. The risk of self-harm may be correspondingly high. Admission—perhaps for only 2 to 3 days— may be indicated in these cases. The risk in major depression is early in the illness or during increasing restlessness after a period of retardation.

2. *Alcoholism and other substance abuse.*

3. *Schizophrenia.* The commonest symptom in schizophrenia is depression.

4. *Early dementia,* perhaps because of brief periods of insight into failing capabilities, or associated with the process.

5. *Epilepsy.*

6. *Following head injury.*

7. *Personality disorder.*

Evaluation of the risk of further self-harm is clearly an inexact process, with weighting of the factors associated with increased risk inevitably seeming arbitrary and not directly applicable to the individual case. Various check lists and rating scales have been devised which are useful to ensure that important questions have been asked, but they must not be accepted as a substitute for an adequate interview, as questions relevant to the individual may be missed. If the patient is aware of the use of a questionnaire to gain important information this may merely distance the patient from the interviewer.

In practice evaluation is concerned with three decisions:

1. To admit to in-patient care.
2. To discharge directly from the A & E department.
3. To allow or arrange for discharge from in-patient care.

1. Few hospitals have special units for the treatment and assessment of patients after the initial physical examination and immediate treatment, and admissions are usually accepted on general medical wards. The requirements for psychosocial assessment (q.v.) almost invariably dictate that a patient should be admitted even if the physical damage (existing or foreseen) is slight and does not require in-patient treatment or observation. Particular aspects supporting admission are:

a. continuing suicidal ideas;
b. living alone;
c. presentation at night alone;
d. when full assessment is not possible;
e. first episode of deliberate self-harm;
f. risk factors (above).

2. To discharge directly from A & E department:

a. This may be a temptation or result from a desire not to reinforce the repetitive self-poisoning or self-mutilating behaviour of a small group of 'chronic repeaters', but these cases are at risk statistically of eventual suicide and each instance should be assessed and treated in the normal way unless a specific treatment programme is in operation (*see* Note 4 on p. 175 later in this chapter).

b. Direct discharge may be possible if:

  i. there are no significant physical problems;
 ii. information has been obtained from friends or relatives and someone will accompany the patient and remain with him at home;
iii. the act was impulsive and repetition is judged to be unlikely by the patient and interviewer;
 iv. ideas of suicide are absent;
  v. the assessement has been adequate and factors indicating increased risk are absent.

A past psychiatric history of itself is not a contraindication for discharging from the A & E department directly but may indicate that advice be sought from the duty psychiatrist, particularly if the patient has been treated for a psychiatric condition at the hospital; if there is a history of major depressive illness; if there is a doubt about the contribution of chronic mental illness to the episode.

3. To allow or arrange discharge from inpatient care. If discharge is arranged:

a. A friend or relative must be fully informed about the self-harm (with the patient's prior consent), and told of the need for continuous support until an early out-patient appointment is attended (less then one week).
b. The GP should be informed by telephone on the day of discharge or the next morning.

Sometimes the patient will want to leave the medical ward before either further medical attention (for example in the treatment of paracetamol poisoning) or an adequate psycho-social assessment has been achieved. In either case if there is felt to be a risk efforts must be made to persuade the patient to stay; it may be helpful to involve friends or relatives. Persuasive powers vary but it is helpful to indicate by attitude that the patient is worth helping and that a few days in hospital could help and is unlikely to result in any overall loss to the patient. The time which needs to be spent on persuasion is arbitrary but anything less than 20 minutes could be considered perfunctory.

Compulsory detention cannot be employed to treat a physical condition alone (e.g. a patient refusing methyl-cysteine for paracetamol poisoning). If gastric lavage is refused the known risk of omitting this has to be balanced against the hazards of lavage in a resisting patient. In an emergency any physical treatments can be given if this would be the practice of a competent doctor acting reasonably (judged by peers). The grounds for compulsory detention are discussed in detail in Chapter 20. Most problems relating to a refusal of treatment can be avoided by careful explanation of the reasons for that treatment, before it is attempted. Arrangements for discharge from hospital should follow a plan of treatment.

## TREATMENT AND AFTER CARE

Most of those who attend hospital after deliberate self-poisoning are young (less than 35) and have taken an overdose with mixed motives (which may have included a wish to die at the time) in the setting of marital, family or other personal conflict. Most of these do not repeat the act although a proportion develop into 'chronic repeaters' (see Note 4 on p. 175 below).

In many of those surviving after deliberate self-harm the common symptoms of depression, anger, and a feeling of hopelessness are more a reflection of psychological distress than of major psychiatric syndromes. A significant number will have long-standing personality traits which interfere with the development of stable relationships and predispose towards symptoms of anxiety and depression. Difficult social circumstances may well compound the problem, with the ability to cope finally undermined with resort to minor tranquillisers and perhaps with the disinhibiting or depressive effects of alcohol and an episode of self-poisoning.

The accepted rationale for treatment is that suicide or self-harm is undesirable and should be prevented if possible, and that immediate treatment is required to respond to the distress associated with the aftermath of most episodes of self-harm. Where there is serious mental illness the priority is for specialist care, probably as an in-patient, but for the majority of patients the principles guiding the provision of help are common to any counselling or crisis intervention service (q.v.). Current personal (marital, difficulties with children) and general (financial, housing) problems need to be discussed with the patient.

It is not the task of the interviewer to convince the patient that life is worth living but rather to help the patient recognise that failure to cope can arise from common problems which can become overwhelming if faced unsupported or where there is rejection. Listing current problems with the patient, dividing these into those which are irreversible (divorce, loss of a particular job, bereavement) and into those which can be influenced, even if only slowly in stages, can be a therapeutic measure, replacing feelings of helplessness with those of increased control.

The proccess of assessment itself can be perceived as beneficial by the patient. Few people have the opportunity to talk in such an open way about their worries and personal difficulties and this can bring release from previously hidden feelings.

Appropriate treatment may range from the assessment and

one or two out-patient appointments to intermittent support over many years in more seriously disturbed individuals.

There are two important points to remember:

1. In some instances where there is evidence of consistent and helpful support from within the family or from friends, it may be more constructive for any professionals involved to reinforce this help and limit their own contact to a post-discharge out-patient appointment or refer back to the GP.
2. Patients who refuse treatment, admission, or leave prematurely may be particularly at risk. It can be helpful to have an arrangement with the department of psychiatry so that an appointment card can be offered for an out-patient appointment—either with a specific time, if this can be arranged, or for a particular out-patient clinic. This link may be sufficient to prevent a recurrence of the self-harm.

## NOTES

### 1. CONTINUITY OF ASSESSMENT AND TREATMENT

One of the problems of admission to hospital after self-harm is that the patient may be seen and assessed by a number of doctors and possibly other (non-medical) staff. It may not be possible for the admitting doctor on the medical unit at night to see the patient to obtain a full assessment on the next day. Certainly this doctor is unlikely to be involved in later treatment. Such fragmentation of care cannot foster the necessary alliance with the patient unless there is adequate explanation of the relative roles of those in contact with the patient at that time. A clear policy needs to be developed covering treatment in the A & E department, and on the medical wards.

## 2. REFERRAL TO A PSYCHIATRIST

This topic is covered in more detail in Chapter 2. A brief formulation including information about past psychiatric history, the reason for referral and clinical urgency is necessary. Conversations such as the following occur more often than is desirable.

*Case example:* Casualty officer to duty psychiatrist: 'Please could you see this patient at once; she doesn't want to stay/is threatening to leave.' Duty psychiatrist: 'Can you tell me what her problem is, please?' 'She's cut her wrists.' 'Is she suicidal, a patient of this hospital, alone. . .?' 'We're very busy, I haven't the time to ask. . . .'

Clearly, if the casualty officer and duty psychiatrist are unknown to each other both may be becoming exasperated. The casualty officer has to decide on priorities, the patient is 'obviously' psychiatric and the pressure of work in the A & E department is unpredictable. The psychiatrist feels entitled to a standard of referral that may be accorded to other specialists, also needs to assign priorities, may need to check in the records department, cannot physically prevent a determined, uncooperative patient from leaving the hospital any more successfully than the A & E staff, and, initially at least, has less information than the casualty officer if use of the Mental Health Act 1983 is contemplated. The patient's interest is paramount, and nothing is achieved—and indeed something may be lost—if the above interchange continues. In practice the casualty officer should be able to form a reasonably accurate assessment but if he cannot, perhaps because the patient is uncommunicative, then one has to accept that individuals who harm themselves and then refuse to accept help that is offered, even if adequate explanation is given for any delay, put themselves at risk, and beyond the immediate help or responsibility of the medical and other staff.

In the above case, the psychiatrist could ask the casualty

officer to sit briefly with the patient, or get another member of the staff to do so, and suggest that the patient stays until the psychiatrist arrives (an estimated time of arrival should be given). If the patient insists on leaving and there appear to be no grounds for detention under the Mental Health Act the patient should be given an appointment to be seen within 1–2 days, and the GP informed. Inform the police if there are threats to other people. Direct physical restraint or sedation is rarely justified.

### 3. ATTITUDES OF STAFF TOWARDS PEOPLE WHO DELIBERATELY HARM THEMSELVES

The treatment of the patient's physical condition should not exclude an appropriate psychological response and good practice would, as far as possible, include simultaneous consideration of physical and psychological factors. At minimum this would involve an uncensorious attitude and explanation, particularly if more urgent cases prevent the unhurried interview required. Negative feelings within the health service towards people who harm themselves deliberately (or abuse drugs or alcohol) are documented. It is worth considering that apart from possible logical inconsistencies in relation to other conditions which are treated without such a reaction in hospital, a critical attitude may make it more difficult to elicit information relevant to making decisions about the patient.

*Negative attitudes* (mainly rejection) can arise from:

a. *Projection of moral values* (feeling that patients should adhere to certain moral imperatives) onto the patient with a resultant disdain for perceived weakness or lack of responsibility. It is only within the past 30 years that attempted suicide has ceased to be a criminal offence, and certain religions consider suicide to be sinful.

b. *Personal anxiety* arising from: (i) an inability to deal with a mute and otherwise uncooperative patient whose attitude may be quite dissimilar to patients admitted for other reasons; (ii) concern about responsibility for the patient if he cannot be persuaded to stay or accept treatment; (iii) a possible need to physically restrain the patient with doubts about how hard to struggle if the need arises.

c. *A loosely formed set of values* about the deference due to doctors and nurses, and the place of deliberate self-harm in a hierarchy of less deliberate (perhaps chronic) self-harm resulting in trauma or acute or chronic illness (sporting injuries; smoking).

A combination of these factors can give rise to punitive and other aggressive feelings from which the patient should be protected. Even if disdain and a strictly not necessary lavage were effective in reducing self-poisoning, the ethics of such management are clearly questionable in medical practice.

## 4. 'CHRONIC REPEATERS'

The permanent staff of every A & E department and psychiatric unit will become familiar with a number of individuals who repeatedly deliberately poison or cut themselves. Frustration can arise in staff because no approach seems to affect the behaviour or the patient's ability to cope with stress and upset in a different way. Such patients tend to have a disorganised life-style often associated with abuse of alcohol and drugs and may suffer from long-standing disorders of personality including sociopathy. They have an increased risk of suicide but may eventually become more stable socially. Each case of self-harm should be treated on its merits unless a particular approach to treatment has been agreed with the patient and all involved staff. Frustration can be reduced if staff accept that significant improvement may be unrealistic in this small number of often highly disturbed individuals and that simply keeping the patient alive by necessary treatment and support may be the limit of that which can be achieved in the short term.

It is difficult to be sure whether attitudes of staff or the supportive regimes presently offered reinforce this behaviour or inhibit a change which would benefit the patient. One could suggest that disdain—whether by rejection or by undue familiarity; 'It's June again, . . . What do you want this time, June?'—may aggravate the syndrome by reducing self-esteem.

### 5. PATIENTS WHO APPEAR TO HAVE BEEN BANNED FROM THE HOSPITAL PSYCHIATRIC UNIT AND WHO IN NORMAL PRACTICE WOULD BE ADMITTED

In practice such a ban cannot be applied since mental state is unpredictable. Usually the patient is one who has a severe disorder of personality with or without other psychiatric diagnoses, and who in the past has not complied with advised treatment and may have been violent towards staff or caused considerable disruption and hazard to other patients when admitted. If in doubt, the consultant psychiatrist on call should be contacted or the patient admitted overnight (with the nursing staff involved in the decision) for assessment the following day. If the patient is outside the hospital and advice is being sought on management, the consultant or senior registrar on call should be involved in case it is appropriate to see the patient in the surgery/police station/home.

### 6. YOUNG PEOPLE

a. *Children.* Self-poisoning with intent of harm or suicide is rare in children and it is usual for health districts to have a specific policy of admission to a children's unit in every case of self-poisoning, including apparent accident poisoning. There is an association between adult self-poisoning and physical abuse of their children and problems such as this may not be elicited or be denied. Where no understandable reason for the episode of self-harm emerges from the assessment interview, the possibility of more serious personal problems should be considered. Rare, but important not to miss, are presentations of illness or injury in children which are factitious—being produced by the parent or carer (Polle syndrome, Munchausen by proxy). The parent will often have a psychiatric history.

b. *Adolescents.* Sometimes in adolescents depression and poor self-esteem may be masked by an alienating irritability or compensatory arrogance with bridling under the authority of an articulate, confident interviewer, or there may be a sullen disinclination to say anything. A younger or very much older interviewer may be successful in relating in these cases.

## 7. THE ELDERLY

This group is at particular risk of eventual suicide. Suggestions that the patient was muddled or took the tablets accidentally under other circumstances should never be accepted without supporting evidence from the assessment and an independent informant.

## 8. SELF-MUTILATION

This refers to the superficial cuts, commonly on the wrists and arms of patients, which are usually inflicted without suicidal intent but to relieve intolerable dysphoria. There are often no clear precipitating events. The act appears to be carried out quite coolly without the experience of serious pain and is followed by relief and relative calmness. Where the act is repetitive, and the patient known, in most instances admission is not indicated or requested and simple treatment of the injury with GP follow-up is all that is required. This type of injury has to be distinguished from more serious injuries close to vital points with suicidal intent. There are often severe problems of personality and self-laceration may be associated with impulsive, aggresive behaviour and drug and alcohol abuse. Sometimes laceration occurs in borderline personality or schizophrenic patients when there are disturbances of body image and the pain produced can be seen as a way of trying to remain in contact with reality (to prove the presence of feelings).

## 9. PSYCHIATRY AND THE A & E DEPARTMENT

Regular contact with the A & E department by the senior registrar or a designated consultant in psychiatry to discuss approaches to particular patients, the feelings these patients arouse, and the service provided by the duty psychiatrists at SHO and registrar level should be, but rarely is, provided. This is especially desirable where the A & E department does not have a consultant in charge. Departments which automatically refer all 'psychiatric' cases without assessment are not providing essential training in dealing with psychiatric emergencies and may foster an attitude which will be particularly inappropriate for those entering general practice. It is arguable that the recommended system does ensure that the chances of missing those at serious risk and of failing to provide the required support are reduced.

*Case example:* A 35-year-old single woman living alone presented with lacerations to both forearms requiring 30 sutures, which she then pulled out . She had a past history of repeated admissions to the psychiatric unit, with episodes of violence towards staff and non-compliance with treatment for abuse of minor tranquillisers and alcohol. She suffered from repeated dysphoria in the setting of a severe personality disorder. She had numerous scars from previous lacerations in addition to new wounds. On presentation she was mildly intoxicated but otherwise physically fit. She was intermittently abusive and uncooperative. She denied suicidal intent and felt less tense than before cutting herself. She did not wish to come into hospital, and could offer no explanation for her actions. On discussion with the responsible consultant it was found that she had been functioning reasonably well when seen in out-patients the previous week.

Her behaviour and bizarre relationship with the accident and emergency department were not understandable except generally in terms of the chaotic drives and personal motivation seen in the more serious disorders of personality (q.v.). That only limited treatment can be offered has to be accepted in these rare cases. Compulsory admission is not indicated, and the patient should be followed up in the outpatient clinic.

## RATIONAL SUICIDE

Sometimes an individual will present with terminal illness, or following severe incapacitating injury, or living a lonely and isolated life when elderly, without the usual accompaniments of depressive illness apart from the conviction that life is not worth living and the future holds no worthwhile prospects. The interviewer may well wonder if he might not feel the same way in similar circumstances.

As noted earlier occasional thoughts about life not being worthwhile are common, but a coherent, controlled individual whose history and mental state do not indicate mental illness together with evidence of carefully arranged plans for suicide which went astray (perhaps because of the chance call of a relative) presents a problem for the interviewer requiring skill and experience. Such a patient represents a serious suicidal risk, but how far is one entitled to interfere?

The immediate practical step is that the patient should remain in hospital until he has had the opportunity to speak to an experienced counsellor. Attitudes to life and suicide vary and touch upon questions of value which few have confronted in their own lives. The working hypothesis is that such a patient needs to talk, and until demonstrated otherwise his suicidal ideas and rationalisations are a defence for a psychological disturbance of which he may be wholly or partly unaware. While it may appear that in his rationalisation he is seeking agreement from the interviewer, to agree that his situation is indeed hopeless may be suddenly devastating and precipitate the suicide.

Could such a person be detained under the Mental Health Act (q.v.)? The wording of the act is sufficiently vague for the answer to be yes; such a course of action is undesirable, and should be unnecessary if skilled and experienced personnel are available to interview the patient.

## CONCLUSIONS

Individual instances of self-poisoning or other self-harm are unique, with a complex mixture of personal factors and events contributing to the act, and the prognosis 'just another overdose' is a mistaken and inappropriate response. In the majority of cases, where a mental disorder is absent, brief outpatient follow-up using crisis intervention techniques (q.v.) is the most appropriate treatment.

# 17. Alcohol and drug abuse

This chapter is concerned with the effects of chemicals which when ingested alter perception and influence behaviour by acting on the central nervous system: specifically alcohol, barbiturates and other sedative hypnotics, opioids, amphetamines, hallucinogens and solvents.

Symptoms may arise from acute intoxication, withdrawal or irreversible damage of the brain developing from chronic excessive exposure to the drug. It is doubtful whether a convincing distinction can be made between the concepts of *psychological* and *physical dependence* in humans or that these are useful ideas in practice. Symptoms which consistently follow the abrupt cessation or ingestion of some of these chemicals may be unpleasant and herald dangerous physical consequences—although danger is not necessarily related to the intensity of symptoms of withdrawal.

*Craving* is an unhelpful term, since the desired outcome of taking a drug is a reduction, an increase, or a change in particular physical and psychological experiences. This state can be achieved by the use of one substance familiar to the habituee but if the same result could be obtained from another drug the patient will for the moment be satisfied. There is also considerable satisfaction and social reinforcement to be obtained from any ritual revolving around the use of drugs, or from the pleasure that may accompany the appreciation of differences between drugs from various sources, or from the search for an ever better experience. Such factors need to be considered in the long-term management of drug abuse. It is part of the treatment of drug abusers presenting as emergencies to consider the most appropriate form of continuing help whether or not the patient is to be admitted.

Some psychiatrists consider that substance abuse can be a form of self-medication which improves functioning in some individuals. There are parallels with states arising in other behaviour—for example persistent exposure to significant danger in recreational or professional pursuits (climbing, diving, voyeurism), gambling, or sexual activity. Societies (including their systems of law) differ in attitudes towards these activities and substance abuse partly for historical reasons, by chance, and probably by neglect arising from the difficulty of applying rational and acceptable universal standards. Accepting this can help to avoid judgements which may otherwise colour the therapeutic approach to a particular patient.

## CLASSIFICATION OF MENTAL DISORDER ARISING FROM SUBSTANCE ABUSE

The DSM-III classification uses three broad categories for most substances:

1. *Substance induced organic mental disorders:* intoxication, withdrawal syndromes, hallucinatory and paranoid states, for example.
2. *Substance abuse*—behaviourally defined.
3. *Substance dependence*—behaviourally defined.

Thus alcohol abuse is defined by

a. a pattern of pathological alcohol use (further described);
b. impairment in occupational or social functioning;
c. duration of disturbance at least one month.

There is a sub-classification recording the course of the condition (continuous, episodic, in remission, course unknown or first signs of illness with course uncertain).

There are few psychiatric emergencies associated with substance abuse, but the demarcation between psychiatric and other medical conditions is an artefact which should not interfere with the patient receiving (and perceiving) continuous assessment and care. Although aspects relevant to each of the drugs noted above will be discussed under separate headings, emergency presentations by substance abusers may have common features.

1. *Behaviour,* which may be loosely described as 'disturbed'—arousal, distractability, anger or frank hostility, fear.
2. *Psychosis,* with delusional (persecutory) ideas or hallucinatory experiences, the appearance being of an acute schizophrenic illness.
3. Absence of an accompanying friend or relative.
4. An *appearance* suggesting self-neglect and social decline—the stereotype drifting inebriate—provoking obvious distaste in other patients and (often) staff.

Training, often unrealistically, aims at changing staff feelings towards patients perceived as unattractive rather than promoting (more easily achieved) changes of behaviour, which may well be followed by a shift in feelings as treatment becomes more rewarding.

Therefore:

1. *Consider multiple causation* for disturbed or psychotic behaviour in those presenting in an apparently intoxicated condition—particularly if no history is available from a third party.
2. *Avoid stereotyping* or assumptions from regular presentations. Remedial physical illness or changes in mental state may be missed if examination becomes cursory.
3. *Recognise* that substance abuse may be a form of self-medication for depression or intractable problems.

## ALCOHOL

Alcohol is implicated in a high proportion of cases presenting at the A & E department with physical injuries from accidents, fights, and assaults. It is associated with depression and suicidal behaviour and a range of physical complications including acute gastrointestinal disorders.

## INTOXICATION

The most common presentation of abuse of alcohol is acute intoxication. Lack of awareness or a degree of anaesthesia may result in a failure to mention injury or mask the usual signs of fracture or head injury. There is always a danger that if the individual is not cooperative, the physical examination may be insufficiently thorough to identify other medical conditions.

Examination may also reveal:

1. Irritability, loquacity, disturbances of perception— attention, thinking, judgement and emotional control —are associated with intoxication, and will interfere with obtaining an adequate history. It is easy for staff to develop a rejecting and punitive attitude to those viewed as 'old customers'. A calm, uncensorious attitude and the recognition that even brief contact may help (and is unlikely to foster any more dependence on the unit than a peremptory dismissal) is required.

2. Other conditions which may mimic or can be associated with intoxication with alcohol. These include: head injury, hypo/hyperglycaemia, epilepsy (temporal lobe), other intoxicated states caused by drugs used to control epilepsy such as barbiturates and benzodiazepines, and (rarely) cerebellar ataxia and multiple sclerosis.

If a coherent history is not likely to be obtained and there is no relative or friend who can provide information, the patient should be asked to wait until the effects of the alcohol are diminished (aided by tea or coffee).

## PRESENTATIONS OF INTOXICATION WITH ALCOHOL

1. *Intoxicated and troublesome.* Violent and disruptive behaviour cannot be tolerated in hospital and if all reasonable

measures to understand and deal with an individual's problems are taken (Chapters 1 to 3) and the aggressive behaviour continues with risk to the staff and other patients, the assistance of the police may have to be sought. It can be dangerous to use further sedative drugs if the patient is intoxicated and a clear history has not been obtained. In the circumstances described it is an acceptable risk for containment to be arranged by the police, who have access to medical treatment (police surgeon).

2. *A rare idiosyncratic reaction to alcohol* has been described where ingestion of a relatively small amount of alcohol causes agitation, belligerence and the appearance of severe intoxication. This behaviour is atypical when the individual is not drinking. A third party history is important. It may be associated with a previous history of head injury, encephalitis, or severe disorders of personality. The patient should be admitted and subsequently warned of the sensitivity. Drugs taken for allergies and the minor and major tranquillisers and antidepressants may predispose to increased intoxication for a given amount of alcohol.

3. *Intoxicated and demanding admission* for help with alcoholism. Here it is essential to distinguish the medical (including psychiatric) indications for in-patient treatment from other issues which may include:

a. judgements on relative priorities;
b. reservations on admission of chronic or 'revolving door' patients who are for various reasons unrewarding to treat;
c. the setting of conditions for treatment;
d. malingering.

All these may involve rationalisations relating to shortage of admission beds or pessimism over the outcome of admission (perhaps following previous experience of premature discharge, failure to comply with treatment regimes or continued drinking on the wards). Some would argue that motivation for treatment should be demonstrated by the patient attending when sober, others that it is appropriate to admit on request and aim to promote the persistance of the initial resolve to achieve abstinence.

Guidelines for a particular hospital or unit are helpful in using a detoxification service to the best advantage and individual agreements with patients have some value as long as all staff likely to be involved know of the arrangements. This does not alter the requirement to judge each case on its merits on every presentation.

Alcohol withdrawal (below) may occur when the amount of alcohol consumed is reduced but not necessarily stopped, but if an individual is intoxicated to the extent of impaired gait and slurred speech serious withdrawal symptoms are unlikely for at least 24 hours, so the patient can usually be offered help as an out-patient by being offered either:

a. Carbamazepine 200 mg t.d.s. three days supply plus advice to remain abstinent or gradually reduce alcohol consumption with an out-patient appointment within two days; or

b. Referral to the GP who can request an out-patient appointment and perhaps supply drugs to cover staged withdrawal in the meantime.

4. *Intoxicated and threatening suicide.* Particularly in the case of new patients assessment can be difficult in the absence of information from a third party and the safest course may be to admit overnight if there is evidence of depression and suicidal intent, with further assessment next morning.

5. *Intoxicated and suspicious, or where there is evidence of other mental illness.* This may reflect an underlying paranoid psychosis which will be revealed on further questioning. This could arise from organic mental disorder including alcoholism, the use of other chemicals as well, or from a schizophrenic illness with alcohol used to relieve unpleasant symptoms (for example abusive auditory hallucinations). It is

very difficult to assess the degree of mood elevation in a hypomanic patient who is intoxicated—where again alcohol may be taken for self-medication—and admission is often advisable.

## INTOXICATION AND THE LAW

Although drunkenness in a public place is an offence, the futility of invoking the law except in the protection of others (and perhaps the offender) is recognised, and rather than charging individuals the practice of taking them to detoxification centres is generally established in those few areas where such centres exist. Imprisonment is no longer a possible sanction for the offence of being drunk and disorderly. There may be imprisonment for non-payment of fines. On occasion (*see* above) the assistance of the police may be required if there is difficulty in dealing with an individual who is 'drunk and disorderly'; sometimes just the presence of the police will enable sufficient contact to be made with an intoxicated patient to render further action (custody) unnecessary.

## WITHDRAWAL FROM ALCOHOL

Symptoms of withdrawal may be present after about eight hours following abrupt cessation of chronic heavy drinking (half bottle spirits/four Carlsberg Specials daily) or a week of 'binge' drinking (continuously heavily intoxicated). The diagnostic criteria (DSM-III) for alcohol withdrawal are:

Coarse tremor of the hands, tongue and eyelids, and at least one of the following:

1. nausea and vomiting
2. malaise and weakness
3. autonomic hyperactivity (tachycardia, sweating, elevated blood pressure)

4. anxiety
5. depressed mood and irritability
6. orthostatic hypotension

not due to any other physical or mental disorder. At this stage the individual is alert and aware, with tremulousness the main symptom.

All symptoms listed above may develop in the absence of treatment and last for several days before slowly resolving. In some cases there may be progression to withdrawal seizures, hallucinosis and delirium ('delirium tremens'). Delirium usually manifests itself 3 to 5 days after withdrawal of alcohol, so if a patient has been admitted with clear symptoms of withdrawal discharge before 5 days is clinically unsound. The characteristics of delirium arising from the withdrawal of alcohol are not distinguishable from other organic states of delirium (q.v.) but, by reputation, the former is associated with a high mortality (10%). Dehydration, disturbance of electrolytes, and seizures are possible complications. Hypoglycaemia may occur. Inhalation of vomitus with the development of pneumonia is always a risk. Delirium always requires in-patient treatment with full medical support.

*TREATMENT OF ALCOHOL WITHDRAWAL*
Withdrawal from alcohol can be achieved as an out-patient, preferably with daily prescriptions of an appropriate sedative (*see* below), to avoid overdose or misuse. This is likely to be difficult where social support is absent or there is lack of adequate accommodation—circumstances leading to further depression or a sense of hopelessness with resort again to alcohol.

It is clearly easier to achieve detoxification as an in-patient and the general principle is one of sedation, achieved by regular oral medication, using a decreasing regimen not extending usually beyond about 10 days. This should be commenced when there are clear signs of withdrawal (*see* above) or when the individual becomes sober if initially intoxicated and there is reason to suspect prior heavy drinking but withdrawal symptoms have not yet developed. 'As required' medication (unless additional to a withdrawal regime) is unjustified on medical grounds if a withdrawal syndrome has been identified or is likely. The use of minimal amounts of medication so that relief from withdrawal symptoms is also minimal as a reminder of the folly of alcohol abuse is not only unlikely to deter the patient from further drinking but also raises a number of ethical issues including the obligation to provide the most effective treatment.

If the patient develops delirium intravenous diazepam 5 mg every 5 to 15 minutes may be given until calmness is achieved. This requires close monitoring under full medical supervision with facilities to ventilate should respiratory arrest occur. Alternatively an infusion of chlormethiazole may be used, the rate of infusion being 'titrated' against the level of sedation to keep the patient drowsy but awake. Details of the use of such infusions may be found in the British National Formulary. Up to 50–100 mg chlordiazepoxide may be given every hour orally until severe restlessness has resolved. The complications mentioned earlier must be anticipated. If there is lack of response, haloperidol (10–20 mg orally q.d.s.) may be prescribed although this dosage is likely to require concomitant use of an anti-parkinsonism drug such as procyclidine (5 mg b.d. initially), which can also be given i.m. or i.v. Phenothiazines such as chlorpromazine reduce seizure threshold and the postural hypotension often induced make them unsuitable for use in someone likely to be restless and attempting to walk.

*USE OF VITAMINS*

Chronic alcoholism may lead to depletion of thiamine (vitamin B1) due to poor diet or malabsorption, with damage to the CNS precipitating Wernicke's encephalopathy. If there is evidence for severe neglect or delirium intravenous thiamine (50 mg) should be given before infusion of glucose or offering food (failure to do this could further deplete remaining stores of thiamine—possibly worsening the patient's condition). A 6-day course of vitamin B and C injections to all patients undergoing detoxification is probably prudent.

*Case example:* A 55-year-old man was admitted in a state of collapse following perforation of his duodenal ulcer. He was dirty and unkempt and smelt of alcohol. He was operated on as an emergency and 3 litres of dextrose saline were infused post-operatively. After he regained consciousness he was confused, ataxic and confabulating. Intravenous parenterovite produced some improvement, but he sustained a permanent and total loss of his ability to remember new information.

## USE OF ANTICONVULSANTS

1. Seizures may occur during withdrawal at any time—usually within 2 to 3 days of stopping alcohol intake. They are usually brief and generalised—grand mal in form—and rarely progress to status epilepticus. Asymmetry clearly suggests a focal lesion revealed by the lowered threshold for seizures. Post-ictal confusion should resolve several hours after the short period of unconsciousness, otherwise the onset of delirium should be suspected. The use of anticonvulsants is controversial—in a patient who is likely to default then simultaneous cessation of alcohol and anticonvulsant may increase the risk of seizures. Diazepam is probably the most effective drug—given i.v. to control fits.

2. The use of carbamazepine as a drug to reduce the risk of seizures during either in- or out-patient withdrawal has been described. A dosage of 200 mg q.d.s. reducing gradually over 7 days can be prescribed. There are advantages in that the drug does not have some of the undesirable potential for misuse that characterise benzodiazepines.

## WERNICKE'S ENCEPHALOPATHY

Ophthalmoplegia, ataxia and a global confusional state with confusion and memory loss are the most prominent features of an acute syndrome arising from thiamine deficiency and may be iatrogenic if nutrition is attended to before vitamin replacement is given (*see* above). Recognition of the condition may be missed since the classical signs are not invariably present and the onset of symptoms may be gradual over days—or mental 'sluggishness' being the only sign. Wernicke's encephalopathy is a *medical emergency*, potentially reversible, avoiding the permanent memory and other deficits of Korsakoff's psychosis (alcohol amnestic disorder) character-ised by retrograde amnesia and an inability to retain new information. It is treated with intravenous thiamine (above) and other measures as necessary for treatment of delirium (q.v.).

## BARBITURATES

Until replaced largely by the benzodiazepine group of drugs, barbiturates were widely prescribed as hypnotics. Pre-scription outside hospital is now rare but they may be employed in cases of severe intractable insomnia. Young people using barbiturates to achieve intoxication and euphoria or older people abusing prescribed barbiturates to relieve tension and improve ability to cope with stress may be at risk of intoxication or a withdrawal syndrome. Barbiturate usage above 600 mg daily is likely to cause problems if the drug is stopped. Tolerance increases while the toxic dose does not.

1. *Intoxication.* Marked by ataxia and slurred speech without smell of alcohol intoxication (although the two may be combined) and evidence of barbiturate usage.

2. *Withdrawal.* Always requires hospital treatment—may be more severe and lethal than that arising from withdrawal of alcohol; such symptoms as delirium can occur, with seizures, hallucinations, and cardiovascular collapse is possible; management should be on an acute medical ward.
3. *Treatment of withdrawal.* An initial dose of phenobarbitone elixir 200 mg orally 4–6 hourly is used until the patient is comfortable and alert. A daily reduction of 10% or 100 mg phenobarbitone, whichever is the smaller, is then achieved, remaining on a fixed dose for two days if withdrawal symptoms occur. If in-patient detoxification is not possible, a general practitioner may substitute phenobarbitone for the shorter acting substance being abused according to the equivalent table of *Guidelines of Good Clinical Practice in the Treatment of Drug Abuse* (DHSS, 1984) which has been circulated to all UK doctors.

## HEMINEVRIN (CHLORMETHIAZOLE)

This drug is used for detoxification (alcohol) and as a hypnotic for the elderly but routine administration is undesirable because dependence can develop and if abused withdrawal symptoms with seizures and delirium may develop. Hospital admission is then necessary for a gradual withdrawal using chlormethiazole and benzodiazepines. Insomnia and irritability may persist for some months after detoxification.

## BENZODIAZEPINES

There are unlikely to be many psychiatric emergencies related to the abuse of benzodiazepines alone. Intoxication is the most likely presentation with other substance abuse (usually alcohol) involved. Confusion, particularly in the elderly, may arise from muddled compliance with medication or the use of excessive amounts to counter loneliness, anxiety, or insomnia. A withdrawal syndrome may develop in patients who have used even a normal dosage for 3 to 4 months. Anxiety, insomnia, irritability, intolerance of noise, and anorexia may occur several weeks after stopping the drug. Seizures have been reported following abrupt withdrawal. In-patient management is rarely indicated for benzodiazepine withdrawal, and gradual reduction in dosage over 4 weeks is usual. Sometimes the withdrawal symptoms extend over some months; patients require support and explanation with 'a readiness on the doctor's part to accept unusual and prolonged symptoms as withdrawal phenomena, and not as a neurotic over-reaction'.


## OPIOIDS

Opioids may be inhaled as smoke, taken orally, or injected intravenously or subcutaneously. A slang has developed regarding the names or origin of the drugs and their usage. Some doctors may be tempted to show their knowledge of this in an attempt to gain credibility with the patient; a firm but insistent reluctance to be diverted from simple descriptions in plain English of how the drug is used is a better first step in helping the patient face reality and break free from a reinforcing sub-culture. In any case slang is changeable and locally determined so that appropriate use by others is unlikely. There are common presentations to A & E departments:

1. *Simulation of physical illness* usually associated with severe pain for which opioids may be prescribed— e.g. renal colic—in an attempt to obtain admission with the likelihood of receiving opioids at least initially.

Evidence for the illness may be manufactured, e.g. urethral bleeding.
2. *Drug overdose*—intoxication.
3. *Addicts who have developed problems from the therapeutic treatment* of painful disease such as haemophilia, and ask for additional treatment.
4. *Confessed addicts* who have been unable to obtain their regular dosage and are withdrawing or simulate withdrawal symptoms.
5. *Drug related physical conditions.*

## GENERAL PRINCIPLES OF TREATMENT
IMMEDIATE
1. Doctors are largely dependent on patients telling the truth and *cannot reliably detect* those patients who are lying. Thus if there is a reasonable chance that severe pain is being experienced, the patient should be admitted and treated appropriately. In most instances patients' stories are taken on trust, which partially explains the success of a small number of patients to gain short admissions and treatment with narcotics in a large number of hospitals before discovery.
2. Maintenance treatment by long-term prescription of opioids should not be undertaken except in collaboration with a specialist with experience in such treatment. The usual goal is a reducing regime, perhaps after some period of maintenance on a steady dose to enable social or other problems to be dealt with under less stress.
3. Elective admission is advisable in cases where (a) there is marked physical and psychiatric pathology; (b) where there is high daily dosage (greater than 0·5 g diamorphine); (c) there are chaotic or deprived circumstances.
4. There is no indication for a single prescription 'as an emergency' to an unknown addict presenting at the A & E department.

INTOXICATION

Severe opioid intoxication with unconsciousness, marked by pinpoint pupils and shallow respiration, is a medical emergency requiring a narcotic antagonist (Naloxone) and appropriate maintenance of ventilation and blood pressure. Naloxone may cause acute withdrawal.

WITHDRAWAL

Descriptions of the effects of withdrawal from opioids are widely known but generally there is rarely any threat to life or risk of physical damage in the absence of co-existing illness, although there may be disturbance of fluids and electrolytes if anorexia and vomiting occur and are uncorrected by oral replacement. Thus there is no indication for a single prescription of a narcotic such as methadone to an unknown 'addict' presenting as an 'emergency'. It would be reasonable and safe to prescribe one or two doses of a major tranquillizer such as thioridazine (50–100 mg), with a suggestion to obtain referral to a detoxification unit via the GP, or to arrange a routine psychiatric out-patient appointment through the duty psychiatrist.

COCAINE

May be sniffed into the nasal passages or dissolved and injected. The predominant effect is one of stimulation. The user may become garrulous, animated and euphoric.

INTOXICATION

High doses may produce hallucinations—visual, tactile, gustatory, olfactory—and delusions, often with paranoid content. Euphoria may alternate with depression and suicidal ideation. Thus psychiatric symptomatology may mimic that of schizophrenia or manic-depressive psychosis. Physically there may be dilated pupils, hypertension and tachycardia, which lasts for only a few hours (cf. amphetamines). Damage to nasal passages may be evident. If sedation is required major tranquillizers should be used. Treatment of depression may be required if the temptation to use further cocaine to improve depressed mood is to be contained.

## AMPHETAMINES

May be taken by mouth or dissolved and injected. There is some similarity in effect to cocaine. A syndrome similar to that of paranoid schizophrenia may be associated with amphetamine abuse; delirium is also possible. Treatment, if sedation is required, is again by major tranquillizers. Amphetamine withdrawal may involve fatigue, depression with suicidal ideation, and disturbed sleep with increased dreaming.

## CANNABIS

Taken alone this drug is unlikely to provoke symptoms which may be classified as a psychiatric emergency but heavy usage may induce psychosis in those individuals who have an existing (but quiescent) schizophrenic illness. Depression and panic attacks are rarer idiosyncratic responses. Sometimes drugs of the arylcyclohexylamine type (PCP) may be combined with cannabis and smoked together.

## PHENCYCLIDINE (PCP—ANGEL DUST)

Considered in the past as a potential anaesthetic agent. It may be smoked, taken orally, injected or sniffed. Small doses produce a state similar to intoxication with alcohol; higher amounts can produce a dissociative state where the person appears alert but is unresponsive (muteness, no response to non-painful stimuli). Agitation with hallucinations (visual, tactile, auditory) may occur with aggression leading to potential homicide or suicide. Haloperidol is useful in the control of the organic psychosis. The disturbed state may persist for several weeks.

## LYSERGIC ACID DIETHYLAMIDE (LSD)

Perception can be widely disturbed with heightened sensory awareness and change of modality (sounds experienced as colour) with the experience pleasant or disturbing. Delusional beliefs (e.g. of persecution, or of the ability to fly) may have disastrous consequences in isolated cases. Major tranquillizers are used in treatment, sedation being required.

## SOLVENTS

The sniffing of the solvents used in glues, liquid organic cleaning agents, gas from aerosol cans and from lighter gas refills, tends to occur in younger age groups (12 to 16). Intoxication with euphoria and exhilaration and sometimes hallucinatory experiences are achieved; later there are cerebral depressant effects—slurred speech, ataxia and drowsiness. Effects are achieved and fade quickly.

Two common presentations may be anticipated:

1. *The aroused, frightened individual* in whom the use of solvents has induced disturbing changes in perception and behaviour, who may seek help alone or more often be brought by friends.
2. *Parents bringing a child* who has been discovered sniffing glue or inhaling solvents and seeking advice.

Physically there may be erythematous spots around the nose and mouth (from inhalation using a bag) and injection of the conjunctivae. Usually no action is required from the strictly medical point of view, the symptoms resolving rapidly, helped by reassurance. If the sniffing is part of group activity with peers and experimental in nature, low key advice on the hazards (*see* below) of particular practices should be given. If the history suggests chronic usage, severe intoxication, or solitary sniffing, evidence for emotional problems should be sought from the individual and interviewing family members. Solvent abuse may be just one aspect of a pathological response to stress indicating the need for psychiatric intervention. Heavy handed attempts to suppress the behaviour by the family may inadvertently encourage more dangerous practices.

## *PARTICULAR HAZARDS FROM SOLVENT ABUSE*

1. Using a plastic bag over the head with possible suffocation or unconsciousness with inhalation of vomit.
2. Sniffing alone or in dangerous places (cupboards, balconies of flats, etc.).
3. Using pressurised canisters providing greater concentration with loss of consciousness.
4. Combination of solvent sniffing and use of alcohol or other drugs.

## MEDICAL COMPLICATIONS ARISING FROM SUBSTANCE ABUSE

1. *General.* Admission to psychiatric units is inappropriate, mental state alterations being secondary to the physical state. Food may be neglected (particularly with abusers of amphetamines) as a side-effect of the drugs taken or because of opposing financial priorities. Vitamin deficiency may occur. Poor physical state and symptoms assumed to be arising from intoxication or withdrawal may lead to failure of the diagnosis of, for example, septicaemia, hepatitis, or appendicitis. Intoxication may result in injuries being forgotten. Psychological problems may have preceded and also arise from substance abuse.

2. *Respiratory.* Overdose may depress the respiratory centre requiring access to intensive care units. Bronchitis and pneumonia may arise from a combination of poor physical state, suppression of cough reflex, and inactivity. Fillers from tablets crushed and dissolved for injection may accumulate in the pulmonary capillaries.

3. *Cardiovascular.* Attempts at intravenous injection outside the vein may give rise to sterile (filler) or infected abscesses or thrombophlebitis. The latter may eventually lead the chronic abuser to involve veins other than in the arms including femoral and jugular veins. Barbiturates injected by mistake into an artery can cause vasospasm and distal gangrene. Septicaemia should be considered in any drug abuser who is pyrexial. AIDS is a new hazard. Those who have cardiac lesions are at special risk of acquiring subacute bacterial endocarditis, and should be warned that injection is particularly dangerous for them. Abuse of alcohol can cause damage to the muscle of the heart.

4. *Gastrointestinal.* Alcohol may produce gastric irritation and there is an increased incidence of peptic ulceration. Pancreatitis, cirrhosis and alcoholic hepatitis can arise from chronic abuse of alcohol. Hepatitis B may arise from the use of unsterile needles or intimate contact with bodily fluids; 10% of drug users have a positive Australia antigen test (for surface protein antigen).

*Important note:* Accident and emergency staff and psychiatrists who come into contact with drug abusers should discuss with their own pathology laboratory staff or infectious diseases unit procedures for collection of blood samples from patients at risk of carrying hepatitis or suffering from acquired immune deficiency syndrome (AIDS). Ideally a written policy document will be available.

5. *Central nervous system.* In addition to the syndromes described (convulsions, intoxication, delirium, psychosis) permanent damage in the form of dementing illness may

result from abuse of alcohol and cerebellar damage can arise from inhalation of solvents.

6. *Genito-urinary*. The elderly alcoholic may precipitate acute retention if there is prostatic enlargement, with irritability and confusion arising from this rather than directly from intoxication. There is an increased incidence of venereal disease. Although fertility is reduced with irregular menstruation or amenorrhoea with opioid abuse pregnancy is still possible. Pregnant women on opioids should be referred to an obstetrician as a matter of urgency—withdrawal of opioids may cause premature labour, foetal distress or death. Carefully planned post-natal care is essential. Impotence is a well recognised complication of alcohol abuse.

*PITFALLS*

The pressure to obtain drugs or immediate help may involve a proportion of those who contact the medical services in:

   a. exerting considerable emotional persuasion for the doctor to treat them in a way which he feels inappropriate and untherapeutic;
   b. deception—false names and diagnosis (even supported by documentation which appears genuine); the involvement of more than one GP; associates who telephone pretending to be the addict's GP confirming the need for prescription;
   c. theft—of prescription pads, syringes, headed notepaper (drug abusers should never be left alone in a consulting room);
   d. violent or disruptive behaviour.

LEGAL ISSUES

   1. Heroin (diamorphine) and cocaine may not be prescribed for maintenance except by doctors holding a special licence to treat addicts. Any doctor may

prescribe these drugs for the relief of pain whether the patient is abusing the drug or not.

2. The Misuse of Drugs (Notification of and Supply to Addicts) Regulations 1973, require any doctor to notify the Chief Medical Officer of the Home Office in writing within 7 days if he attends a patient whom he considers, or has reasonable grounds to suspect, is addicted to any of the following named drugs: cocaine, dextromoramide, diamorphine, dipipanone, hydrocodone, hydromorphone, levorphanol, methadone, morphine, opium, oxycodone, pethidine, phenazocine, pritramide, papaveretum.

A person is considered to be an addict if, and only if, he has as a result of repeated administrations become so dependent on the drug that he has an overpowering desire for the administration of it to be continued. A casualty officer or duty psychiatrist is unlikely to be sufficiently sure to ascribe the label 'addict' to an unknown patient presenting as an emergency, so unless involved in further assessment will not usually have an obligation to notify as required under the Act (*see* above). It may be useful, however, to enquire to see if the patient has previously been notified as an addict. This can be done by telephoning (between 9.00 and 17.00):

(01) 213 5141 (surnames A–F)
(01) 213 4274 (G–L)
(01) 213 6083 (M–P & S)
(01) 213 6695 (T–Z & QR)

The information in the addicts register is used for providing statistical information and for the information of doctors treating addicts. The Home Office has given an assurance that neither the police forces nor foreign embassies have access to these records.

3. It is not an offence to have or sniff solvents or gases. Under Scottish law children under 16 found sniffing can be referred to the Reporter to a Children's Panel. This could lead to a child being taken into care. It is an offence 'recklessly' to sell solvents to youngsters knowing they intend to misuse them.

## TREATMENT

Treatment should involve consideration of the help likely to be needed in the future by an individual presenting as an emergency. This should include discussion of the agencies available—referral to the local psychiatric unit or drug team should enable appropriate action to be taken—whether direction to rehabilitation houses, in-patient detox, or information centres. Ideally leaflets with such information should be available.

# Part F
# Drugs in emergency psychiatry

# 18. Drug treatment of psychiatric emergencies

In this chapter representative drugs from each major category are discussed from five aspects: indications; contra-indications; side-effects; interaction with other drugs; toxicity and effects of acute withdrawal. Minor side-effects or longer-term side effects are not detailed and reference should be made to the *British National Formulary* (BNF) or the Data Sheet Compendium (produced by the pharmaceutical industry). Toxicity, acute withdrawal, or medium-term side effects may precipitate emergency presentations.

MAJOR TRANQUILLISERS (neuroleptics, antipsychotic agents)

This group of drugs includes phenothiazines (e.g. chlorpromazine) and butyrophenones (e.g. haloperidol). It is helpful to become familiar with the action of just two or three of these compounds so that failure to respond or unusual symptoms can alert the clinician to the need for reassessment of a particular patient. Equivalent doses are given in *Table 18.1*.

*INDICATIONS*
Morbidly high levels of arousal with or without disturbance of behaviour. The aim is to decrease distress and avoid harm, and possibly to initiate continuing treatment. Such states may arise from:

1. *Acute psychoses* (schizophrenia/mania). In catatonia the unresponsive but aroused hypervigilant state may alternate with extremely active, disturbed behaviour which can be lethal (from exhaustion and physiological

*Table* 18.1. EQUIVALENT ORAL DOSES OF PHENOTHIAZINES

| | | |
|---|---|---|
| Chlorpromazine | (Largactil) | 100 mg |
| Thioridazine | (Melleril) | 100 mg |
| Trifluoperazine | (Stelazine) | 10 mg |
| Haloperidol | (Serenace) | 2–5 mg |

complications) and treatment with major tranquillisers should be initiated when this state is recognised (*see* also neuroleptic malignant syndrome below).

2. *Depressive psychosis,* where agitation and distress may arise from delusional beliefs perhaps with the development of paranoid and aggressive behaviour.

3. *Organic brain syndromes,* including dementia, substance abuse, and post-operative confusional states.

4. *Severe anxiety,* where there is panic uncontrollable by verbal support. Major tranquillisers may be more effective than benzodiazepines.

5. *Substance abuse*—symptomatic relief from withdrawal of heroin or other narcotics can be achieved with the use of major tranquillisers.

Information on where further help can be obtained should also be provided together with referral to a psychiatrist (dependent on local policy) or suggestion to contact the GP (or register with a local GP).

## PHENOTHIAZINES

### 1. CHLORPROMAZINE (Largactil)

This drug was synthesized in 1950 by Charpentier, as a relative of known antiparkinsonism and antihistamine drugs. In 1952 Delay and Deniker reported the effects of the drug in the treatment of manic excitement.

The effect is tranquillisation with maintained alertness. Florid psychoses (particularly acute schizophrenia or mania) may require rapid control and chlorpromazine syrup (100 mg) repeated 4-hourly is usual. An initial dose of 150–200 mg will occasionally be desirable for severe arousal. Intramuscular injection (involuntary) is best avoided as this will be perceived as an attack and there is danger of injury to both patient and staff. Intramuscular injection (voluntary) is not justified simply to achieve a more rapid effect; the difference between oral and i.m. routes in clinical response is rarely significant. Where cooperation cannot be achieved i.m. medication may be required but to avoid injury to patient or staff the guidelines discussed under haloperidol for i.v. use should be followed (see below). Marked tranquillizing effects should be obtained within 6 hours.

A daily dosage of 1,000 mg or more may be required in the early stages of treatment. In the elderly the dose required may be considerably less and initially 25–75 mg thioridazine (less likely to cause extrapyramidal side-effects) or promazine (25–100 mg) should be used. This can be repeated and the dosage adjusted 4-hourly as required. Haloperidol is also a useful drug in the treatment of the elderly when used carefully in small doses.

Long-acting (depot) injections should never be used for acute illness, particularly in the elderly, as flexibility of treatment is lost. In known patients with an acute relapse of a psychotic illness it may be appropriate for the psychiatrist responsible to initiate treatment with depot medication at the same time as an oral regime.

## CONTRAINDICATIONS

1. Poisoning caused by CNS depressants (e.g. alcohol or barbiturates).
2. Bone marrow suppression (agranulocytosis is a rare side-effect of chlorpromazine).

3. Cirrhosis or history of jaundice following previous use of chlorpromazine (use alternative, e.g. Stelazine or haloperidol.)

*CAUTION*

1. Elderly and debilitated.
2. Cardiovascular and respiratory disease, Parkinsonism, epilepsy.

*INTERACTION WITH OTHER DRUGS*

Chlorpromazine is compatible with most drugs and the administration of ECT. Liver metabolism of some drugs may be disturbed, usually prolonging their half-life. Extrapyramidal side-effects may be accentuated by metoclopramide.

*SIDE-EFFECTS*

Drowsiness, postural hypotension, blurred vision, dryness of mouth, and mild indigestion.

Patients should be warned of the possibility of hypotension (resting prone after i.m. injections for at least 30 minutes) and asked to get up slowly and walk with care. Stiffness of the limbs (impending dystonic effects or Parkinsonism) should also be reported.

Acute dystonia refers to the sudden development of abnormal movements arising from intense and prolonged muscular contractions, producing torticollis, arching of the back, tongue protrusion, writhing, rolling of the eyes under the lids (*oculogyric crisis*). Sometimes patients may complain of eyelids 'locking' and this is usually a sign that mild dystonic reactions are being experienced, and modification of the drug regime is indicated.

The young are particularly prone to develop these rare but sometimes painful and certainly distressing symptoms. Excessive dosage of the chemically related antihistamines in formulations for cough suppression may provoke an oculogyric crisis in children. Treatment involves the administration of procyclidine (10 mg) either i.m. or i.v. and there is usually a dramatic resolution of the symptoms (within 10 minutes). Diazepam (i.m. or oral) 10 mg (adults) can be used at the same time to relieve anxiety.

Large doses of chlorpromazine can produce indifference to pain (even to fractures) and may mask fever (temperature lowering effect).

In summer there is a serious risk of excessive sunburn due to the photosensitizing effect of chlorpromazine; verbal warning is required and protective cream (mescenone) should be used. In the cold, hypothermia or frostbite of extremities is more likely.

*TOXICITY*

Even large overdoses of phenothiazines (several grammes) are rarely fatal unless taken in combination with other CNS depressants such as alcohol or barbiturates. However, treatment should be on a medical ward with supportive care after lavage. In rare cases hypotension and cardiac arrhythmias can lead to cardiac arrest. Transfer to a psychiatric unit should not occur for three days if doses which are many times normal daily dosage have been taken.

The rare *neuroleptic malignant syndrome* is associated with the administration of major tranquillisers (and the abrupt withdrawal of levodopa in idiopathic Parkinson's disease). An identical syndrome may be seen, again rarely, in untreated catatonic schizophrenia. It may occur hours or months after the last administration of a major tranquilliser. *Rigidity* with bradykinesia and mental withdrawal extending to mutism or catalepsy may occur within one to three days. The dystonia may lead to dysarthria and dsyphagia. *Pyrexia* develops (38·5–42 °C) with sweating and a tachycardia. *Irreversible tissue damage,* leading to cardiovascular, respiratory and renal complications may result in death even with supportive measures.

## 2. HALOPERIDOL

Haloperidol is chemically distinct from the phenothiazines, but has similar effects. When given intravenously haloperidol can be very effective in calming seriously disturbed patients but this technique must only be used in the unwilling patient where there is a need for urgent treatment to avoid harm or injury to the patient or others. At least five helpers are required to restrain the patient with minimal force (*see* Chapter 10). When inadequate help is available no attempt at intravenous injection should be made. The doctor should explain what is about to happen and why as the procedure is carried out. A butterfly infusion needle with flexible connector should be used as movement will be less likely to cause the needle to leave the vein or produce injury. Haloperidol 5–10 mg injection should be followed by procyclidine 10 mg by the same route but in a different syringe.

The most important signs of improvement in mental state are an increasing awareness of staff and surroundings and recovery of social judgement. A total oral daily dose of haloperidol of up to 100 mg (divided) may be required, once control has been achieved. In the elderly confused patient aggression or anxiety may be treated successfully with haloperidol in much smaller doses—initially 0·5 mg b.d. The drug has a greater potential to induce extrapyramidal symptoms than chlorpromazine but cardiac effects are probably less. In depressive psychosis or severe anxiety in younger adults a sedating drug such as chlorpromazine is more appropriate.

### CAUTION

1. Poisoning with CNS depressants (e.g. alcohol and barbiturates).
2. Basal ganglia disease.
3. The elderly—but do not neglect its use as it can be a very

effective drug particularly as the danger of increased confusion from drowsiness is less with haloperidol.

## INTERACTION WITH OTHER DRUGS
1. *See* under chlorpromazine.
2. Caution if the patient is taking lithium—side-effects may be potentiated.

## SIDE-EFFECTS
Less anticholinergic and hypotensive effects than chlorpromazine but dystonic reactions are more likely.


## ANTIPARKINSONIAN DRUGS (anticholinergic type)

These drugs can be used to treat any symptoms of Parkinsonism produced after a patient has been established on major tranquillisers. Drug-induced Parkinsonism is characterized by increasing stiffness of the limbs, cramps, some loss of facial expression (may be mistaken for apathy or depression) and, more rarely, excessive salivation.

## INDICATIONS
Antiparkinsonian agents should only be used when side-effects (dystonia, Parkinsonism) appear. They should not be prescribed routinely; reducing the dose of major tranquilliser should be considered first. The exception to this rule is when haloperidol is given intravenously; procyclidine may then be given at the same time in a different syringe—since extrapyramidal effects are much more likely in these circumstances. The reasons for withholding anticholinergic medication are:

    a. there may be a greater risk of inducing the long-term side-effect of tardive dyskinesia (controversial);

    b. the drugs have their own undesirable side-effects (*see* below);

   c. the early signs of tardive dyskinesia may be masked;
   d. the drug is unnecessary and the initial prescription is regrettably continued in combination with the antipsychotic drug without review.

## PROCYCLIDINE

There may be individual differences in the tolerance to the various anticholinergic drugs, of which procyclidine is an example. Orphenadrine is sometimes favoured for use with the elderly.

The daily dose needed to control extrapyramidal symptoms produced by major tranquillisers is usually not more than 20 mg. This should be given in divided doses (initially 5 mg b.d.). In acute dystonia procyclidine 5 mg i.v. is frequently effective within five minutes. On occasion more than 10 mg and up to 30 minutes may be required before the symptoms are totally relieved; i.m. administration is also effective between 5 and 30 minutes after administration. The drug should then be given orally if the dose of major tranquilliser needs to be maintained.

## CONTRAINDICATIONS

There are no absolute contraindications for treatment of dystonia. The presence of tardive dyskinesia is (controversially) a contraindication.

## CAUTION

1. Predisposition to (closed-angle) glaucoma.
2. Obstructive disease of the gastrointestinal tract—anticholinergic action reduces motility.
3. Prostatic hypertrophy.

## SIDE-EFFECTS

Those to be expected from anticholinergic action are:

1. *Central:* nausea and drowsiness.
2. *Peripheral:* dry mouth, constipation, urinary difficulties.

*TOXICITY*

An acute organic delirium may result with high dosage or abuse, particularly with the elderly. Anticholinergic drugs may also be abused for their stimulating and euphoriant effects.

## OTHER DRUGS USED FOR SEDATION IN THE ACUTELY DISTURBED

*PARALDEHYDE*

There is some distaste for using this drug because of its association (not least by its smell) with the treatment of patients in institutions before modern antipsychotic drugs were available; there are also possibilities of harm when the drug is given by deep intramuscular injection (abscess formation). Paraldehyde is a safe, rapidly acting sedative, excreted predominantly through the lungs. The only clinical use for this drug according to the BNF is for the treatment of status epilepticus. However, it does remain for use in A & E departments and can be helpful in the rare instances where rapid sedation is required to prevent injury to the patient or other people in, for example, psychotic illness. The liquid dissolves plastic so glass syringes should be used.

Paraldehyde can be used orally but is a gastric irritant: the dose is 5–10 ml. A similar dose can be given by deep intramuscular injection but no more than 5 ml should be given at any one site because of the danger of abscess formation and damage to the sciatic nerve.

*CONTRAINDICATION*

If the patient is using Antabuse (disulfiram).

## MINOR TRANQUILLISERS

This misleading term is usually reserved for the benzo-diazepines, a group of compounds used variously as sedatives

*Table* 18.2. EQUIVALENT DOSAGE AND RELATIVE DURATION OF ACTION OF BENZODIAZEPINES

| | *Half-life of active metabolites* | *Daily dosage* |
|---|---|---|
| *Long-acting* | | |
| Diazepam (Valium) | 20–100 hours | 6–30 mg    (60 mg) |
| Chlordiazepoxide (Librium) | 12–24  hours | 30–100 mg  (400 mg) |
| *Short-acting* | | |
| Lorazepam (Ativan) | 12 hours | 2–10 mg |
| Oxazepam (Serenid) | 8–15 hours | 15–180 mg |

for anxiety, as hypnotics, to promote muscle relaxation and as anticonvulsants. Equivalent doses and relative duration of action are given in *Table* 18.2.

## INDICATIONS

Indications in emergency psychiatry are virtually limited to the treatment of withdrawal states (*see* Chapter 17). Morbid levels of anxiety are usually more appropriately treated by psychological measures or, if accompanying psychotic illness, with the use of a sedative major tranquilliser such as chlorpromazine. The use of intravenous benzodiazepine is not recommended for the control of anxiety—there are hazards (*see* below). Giving a benzodiazepine i.v. in the normal way as a pre-medication in ideal conditions is quite different from its use in a patient who may be unable or unwilling to remain supine or still, when there may also be a temptation to administer the dosage too quickly. Severe neurotic reactions including regressive behaviour can respond quickly to oral diazepam (5–10 mg) combined with reassurance.

## DIAZEPAM

This is a benzodiazepine with a relatively long half-life and the usual dosage for moderate anxiety is 2–5 mg given orally twice or three times daily. Larger dosages are appropriate for withdrawal states; chlordiazepoxide may also be used.

## CONTRAINDICATIONS
Acute pulmonary insufficiency or respiratory depression.

## CAUTIONS
1. Use of other centrally acting depressants—alcohol, barbiturates, phenothiazines, etc.
2. In the elderly—particularly those with dementing illness —confusion may be increased with long-acting benzodiazepines.
3. There may be an accumulation of active metabolites.
4. A history of multi-drug abuse.

## INTERACTIONS WITH OTHER DRUGS
Levels of other anticonvulsants may be affected by the presence of diazepam.

## SIDE-EFFECTS
General effects are drowsiness, sedation and ataxia. Rare effects include nausea and headaches. Abnormal psychological reactions have been reported: paradoxical aggressive outbursts, excitement, confusion and depression. Disinhibition may be more likely in those already impulsive by nature (similar to the effect of alcohol).

### INTRAVENOUS USE
Where a decision to use diazepam intravenously is made the following possible side-effects should be considered. The usual dose is 10–20 mg at 4-hourly intervals.

1. *Apnoea and hypotension.* Facilities for resuscitation and mechanical ventilation with supporting staff should be immediately available. Injections should be given slowly (0·5 ml per minute) with the patient in supine

position to the point where the patient is drowsy with slurred speech but can still respond to requests. Someone must remain with the patient for at least one hour after injection.

2. *Local reactions.* Thrombophlebitis and venous thrombosis may be avoided by using the large antecubital vein, slow administration, and a small needle with a flexible connector to the syringe (e.g. butterfly). Use of an emulsion formulation (diazemuls) is preferable.

## TOXICITY

Benzodiazepines have largely replaced barbiturates as sedatives and hypnotics and are rarely fatal in overdose when taken alone; with alcohol or other depressants they may contribute to fatal poisoning. The elderly are particularly susceptible to side-effects and half the normal dosage is advisable initially. In emergency psychiatry there is no indication for the use of short-acting benzodiazepines such as lorazepam and oxazepam.

*Acute withdrawal,* particularly where there has been abuse of the drug, usually occurs within 2–3 days. Tachycardia, tremor, nausea, hallucinations, depression and seizures can be produced, with severe insomnia. Treatment involves reinstatement of a long-acting benzodiazepine with a withdrawal period of up to several months.

## ANTIDEPRESSANTS

The fact that improvement in mood often takes ten to fourteen days to develop once antidepressants have been started is not an argument for delaying prescription when a patient presents with a history and symptoms of biological depression in the A & E department (*see* Chapter 7). In certain circumstances it may be helpful to supply an appropriate antidepressant:

1. if the patient's general practitioner can be consulted and treatment agreed with an early appointment arranged;
2. if the duty psychiatrist agrees and can arrange an appointment within three days.

The advantages of initiating treatment at this stage are:

1. immediate relief of agitation from the sedative action of the antidepressant, with alleviation of insomnia;
2. the psychological value of treatment and follow-up arrangements being arranged at the time help is sought.

The reservations attached to the prescription of anti-depressants in an emergency usually relate to the risk of overdose and attempted suicide (although the potential danger can be reduced by only prescribing three days' supply) and the possibility of non-compliance because of side-effects (*see* Chapter 7).

Antidepressants useful where there is anxiety and agitation include amitriptyline (Tryptizol, Lentizol), dothiepin (Prothiaden), and mianserin (Bolvidon, Norval). Less sedation is produced by imipramine (Tofranil), clomipramine (Anafranil) and lofepramine (Gamanil). Amitriptyline and imipramine are probably the most widely known anti-depressants with proven effectiveness when given in adequate dosage. Too low a dosage is the commonest cause of therapeutic failure.

*INDICATIONS*

Moderate and severe depressive illness (DSM–III major depressive illness—*see* Chapter 7).

*AMITRIPTYLINE*

Initially 50–75 mg daily in divided doses or as a single dose at bedtime (elderly 25–50 mg), increasing to a maximum of 150–200 mg daily.

## CONTRAINDICATIONS

1. Cardiac disease—recovery phase of myocardial infarct, arrhythmias (particularly heart block).
2. Existing treatment with monoamine oxidase inhibitors (MAOIs).

## CAUTION

In patients with a history of urinary retention, prostatic hypertrophy, narrow-angle glaucoma, and epilepsy, or where anaesthesia is required (increased risk of hypotension and arrhythmias).

## DRUG INTERACTIONS

1. *Monoamine oxidase inhibitors* (MAOIs)—potentiation with possible fatal outcome. Fourteen days should elapse after discontinuing a monoamine oxidase inhibitor before a tricyclic antidepressant is prescribed.
2. *Alcohol*—CNS depression increased.
3. *Antihypertensives*—diminished effect.
4. *Digitalis*—increased heart block and ectopic phenomena.
5. *Anticholinergic agents*—additive effects.

## SIDE-EFFECTS

Dry mouth, sedation, blurred vision, constipation, postural hypotension, difficulty with micturition. Some symptoms lessen over 2–3 days and compliance should be encouraged. Driving should be avoided if sedation is prominent.

## TOXICITY

High dosage may produce confusion and transient visual hallucinations. Overdosage can produce severe cardiotoxic effects with tachycardia, arrhythmia, bundle branch block, stupor and coma, and death. Close monitoring of cardiac function for five days is advised. (This has implications for accepting patients onto psychiatric units from medical wards after overdose). Abrupt withdrawal may produce rebound cholinergic symptoms (e.g. nausea, diarrhoea) and anxiety and depression.


## GENERAL PRINCIPLES OF PRESCRIBING

The *British National Formulary* is the most useful source of information for most drugs. If in doubt the manufacturers of a particular drug may be contacted by telephone—most will be able to give rapid, appropriate advice.

### 1. POSSIBILITY OF ABUSE OF MEDICATION

Severe anxiety, depression or psychotic illness are distressing and excess medication may be taken to try and obtain relief, sleep or death, not infrequently with the aid of alcohol. In acute situations drugs should be prescribed in small quantities and if possible tablets should be entrusted to a relative. Mental state must be reviewed frequently. Compliance must never be taken for granted.

### 2. PATIENTS MUST BE WARNED OF SIDE-EFFECTS

   a. Where drowsiness and reduced concentration may be dangerous—for example, in operating machinery (including driving): *benzodiazepines, butyrophenones, phenothiazines.*
   b. Where dry mouth, dizziness, early morning drowsiness may produce non-compliance unless encouragement is given to persist with the medication, particularly over the first few days: *tricyclic antidepresants.*
   c. Particularly warn patient (and relatives) of acute effects and give 2 or 3 antiparkinsonism tablets to use if there is a sudden onset of stiffness or dystonia: *phenothiazines, butyrophenones.*
   d. Always warn against concurrent use of alcohol.

### 3. PREGNANCY

The prescription of drugs in the first and last trimesters should be avoided if possible, to lessen the risk of increased incidence of congenital malformations and compromising the viability of the child at birth. Serious mental illness arising from depression, mania or schizophrenia is clearly potentially hazardous to both mother and child. It may also be distressing to the mother and treatment should ideally be shared between the psychiatrist and obstetrician carefully reviewing the dose of psychotropic medication required for adequate treatment of the mental illness. If the mother is taking opiates or abusing other drugs care will need to be exercised in avoiding too sudden a withdrawal of these drugs from the mother. In breast feeding lithium and diazepam may be contained in sufficient quantities in the milk to significantly affect the baby; this is less important with tricyclic antidepressants and phenothiazines.

### 4. THE ELDERLY

Initial doses of all types of medication should be smaller than those suggested for younger adults. In delirium excessive sedation may increase confusion and haloperidol may be effective. Anticholinergic side-effects are more likely to precipitate urinary retention, constipation and gastro-intestinal problems. The tolerance for related drugs varies widely and unpredictably—it is often well worth the additional effort to gradually adjust the dosages, ensure that the time at which the drug is given is appropriate for the desired response, and to try different drugs until the optimum effect is achieved.

# 19. Drugs that may cause psychiatric symptoms

Drugs used in therapeutic amounts for various medical conditions may affect the mental state. Most drugs at sufficient dosage can cause clouding of consciousness and ultimately delirium. Sometimes withdrawal of the drug may precipitate pscyhiatric symptoms. Any drug which depresses the CNS may cause confusion, particularly in the elderly, and produce secondary suspiciousness or frank paranoid ideation. Details of current and past medication (drugs used formerly may have been kept and subsequently taken in overdose) are an essential part of any psychiatric history. Some classifications of drugs causing psychiatric syndromes group the drugs according to predominant effect (e.g. delirium, other psychotic conditions, disorders of mood or other behaviour) but in practice the non-specific action of drugs and individual susceptibilities confound such divisions. It follows that the rigour with which cause and effect can be established is often low.

The list of drugs considered in *Table* 19.1 is not complete, only the commonest drugs likely to be encountered are included. Those in *italics* are used in psychiatry and may be a cause of emergency presentation.

*Table* 19.1 COMMON DRUGS WHICH MAY CAUSE
PSYCHIATRIC SYMPTOMS

| Drug | Psychiatric symptoms | Comments |
|---|---|---|
| *Amitriptyline* | Confusion, hallucinations, paranoia, elevations of mood | |
| Anticholinergics | *See* amitriptyline | May be abused for euphoric effect |
| Anticonvulsants | Delirium | In overdose |
| Antihistamines | *See* amitriptyline | In overdose |
| Atropine | *See* amitriptyline | May be implicated in post-operative confusion |
| Baclofen | Confusion, visual hallucinations, mood elevation | After withdrawal |
| *Benzodiazepines* | Paradoxical rage or excitement | Rare; may reflect underlying traits |
| Bromocriptine | Confusion, hallucinations | High dosage |
| Cimetidine | Confusion | Elderly, poor renal function |
| Corticosteroids | Any psychiatric syndrome | |
| Digoxin | Malaise, delirium, altered colour vision | High dosage |
| *Disulfiram* | Psychotic symptoms | Rare |
| Fenfluramine | Depression | After withdrawal |
| Isoniazid | Delirium, mood elevation | |
| Levodopa | Delirium, depression | Elderly, prolonged use |
| Methyldopa | Depression, paranoia, hallucinations | |
| Nalidixic acid | Visual disturbance | |
| Pentazocine | Nightmares, hallucinations, anxiety | |
| *Phenelzine* | Delusions, aggression | |
| *Phenothiazines* | Akathisia | |
| Propranolol | Depression | |
| Salbutamol | Psychotic states, agitation, elevated mood | Abuse |
| Sympathomimetics (nasal sprays, cold remedies, anorectics) | Amphetamine-like reactions | |

# Part G
# Legal issues

# 20. Mental illness and the law

Disturbance of mood (hypomania/depression), thinking (involving problems with concentration, memory, organisation), and perception (hallucinatory and delusional experiences or illusional misinterpretation) can affect the behaviour of an individual sufficiently to put at risk his own health or safety or place others in need of protection. The Mental Health Act 1983 is concerned with the grounds for detaining such individuals in hospital to ensure assessment or treatment under medical supervision. These disturbances of mental functioning may be present or have been noted before in persons charged with offences against the law; forensic or general psychiatrists may be asked to express an opinion on the relationship between these symptoms and the offence. The assessment and management of aggressive or violent behaviour is described in Chapter 10.

## MENTAL HEALTH ACT 1983

The Mental Health Act 1983 consolidated the Mental Health Act 1959 as amended by the Mental Health Amendment Act 1982. In essence, a more complex form of legal and medical audit of the treatment of mental disorder both in and outside hospital has been initiated.

### COMPULSORY DETENTION

The compulsory detention of patients in hospital for assessment and treatment can be supported under the Act if *all three* of the following conditions are fulfilled:

1. There is evidence for mental disorder (defined below).
2. The nature of the mental disorder warrants the detention of the patient in hospital for assessment, or for assessment followed by medical treatment (*treatment*

includes 'nursing . . . care, habilitation and rehabilitation under medical supervision') for at least a limited period.

3. The patient ought to be detained in the interests of his health or safety or with a view to the protection of others.

## MENTAL DISORDER

This is defined as 'mental illness, arrested or incomplete development of mind, psychopathic disorder, or any other disorder or disability of mind'. 'Mental illness' is not defined further in the Act, and remains a matter of clinical judgement, but would broadly include categories in the International Classification of Diseases. This is clearly a wide definition and it can be used for implementation of Section 2 (*see* below). A more restrictive definition is used for most purposes of the Act in which the mental disorder must be one of the four categories—mental illness, mental impairment, severe mental impairment, or psychopathic disorder. The term mental impairment replaces the word subnormality in the 1959 Act. Mental impairment is defined as 'a state of arrested or incomplete development of mind which includes significant impairment of intelligence and social functioning', but for the purposes of the Act this must be associated with 'abnormally aggressive or seriously irresponsible conduct'.

(*Note:* 'Section' simply refers to the numbered divisions or 'sections' in the text of the Act. The Sections themselves, are grouped into several 'Parts'; hence the term 'Part III Accommodation' arises from the Part of the Act (1959) referring to Mental Nursing Homes and Residential Homes.)

Psychopathic disorder is defined as a 'persistent disorder or disability of mind (whether or not including significant impairment of intelligence) which results in abnormally agressive or seriously irresponsible conduct on the part of the person concerned'. Persistent implies that the behaviour described was recognisable by the time of adolescence or earlier.

## EXCLUSIONS FROM THE DEFINITION OF MENTAL DISORDER

Section 1(3) of the Act states that a person may not be dealt with under the Act as suffering from mental disorder purely by reason of promiscuity, other immoral conduct, sexual deviance, or dependence on alcohol or other drugs. It is recognised that alcohol or drug abuse may be associated with or accompanied by mental disorder, e.g. intoxication or delirium arising from abuse of alcohol (*see* Chapter 17).

## COMPULSORY DETENTION FOR ASSESSMENT OR TREATMENT OF MENTAL DISORDER

It is important to note that it is not possible to use the Mental Health Act to give medical treatment other than that required for treatment of the mental disorder. Thus the Act cannot be used to force an individual to undergo lavage of the stomach after an overdose of paracetamol or to carry out operative procedures unconnected with the treatment of any mental disorder in a surgical in-patient, who is, however unwisely, refusing the proposed operation.

Only Sections 2, 4, 5(2), 5(4) and 136 are likely to be relevant in emergency psychiatry.

## SECTION 5(2): APPLICATION IN RESPECT OF A PATIENT ALREADY IN HOSPITAL

This section can be applied to a patient already receiving any form of in-patient treatment on a general hospital ward as well as on a psychiatric unit. It cannot be used in the casualty department where the patient is technically an out-patient. It has to be applied by the registered medical practitioner in charge of treatment—usually interpreted as the consultant physician or surgeon (if on a general hospital ward and not currently receiving psychiatric treatment) or (if the patient is receiving psychiatric treatment on the general medical ward) by the consultant psychiatrist providing treatment; one nominated deputy may make the application on behalf of the consultant in his absence. The Section provides that the patient may be detained for up to 72 hours (including any period during which a nurse's holding power—*see* Section 5(4) below—was used).

This allows time for the second recommendation and involvement of relatives or social worker required under Sections 2 and 3. In implementing Section 5(2) the medical practitioner in charge of treatment is reporting that application under Section 2 or 3 should be made.

Where such a report is made by a non-psychiatrist, a senior psychiatrist should see the patient as soon as possible to determine whether further detention is required.

The medical practitioner acting as 'nominated deputy' is determined by local circumstances and his or her identity should be readily available to staff.

USE OF SECTION 5(2)

Sometimes records show that a patient admitted informally to a psychiatric unit is placed on Section 5(2) within one or two days. The Act does not include a refusal to enter hospital informally as a ground for implementation of a Section authorising compulsory detention, but there is a requirement to specify 'why informal admission is not appropriate in the circumstances of this case . . .'. Clearly a refusal would be one reason but another could be that the patient is unable to give a valid consent either to be admitted or to stay—for example consent may be unreliable if the mood is severely disturbed (*see* also Chapter 21).

Does the use of Section 5(2) shortly after admission indicate a failure to appreciate the mental state of the patient or a failure to abide by the spirit of the Act as some suggest?

Can the patient say with some justifiable sense of grievance, 'I agreed to come into hospital of my own accord, but now I am not allowed to go'?

It could be argued that if a patient fulfils the criteria for compulsory admission then the Act should be invoked whether or not the patient agrees to enter the hospital informally. However, the primary purpose of the Act is to enable a patient to receive medical assessment and treatment and therefore if the patient enters the hospital having given consent which is likely to be unreliable (in the sense that a change of mind may come about) this is not of importance until that patient wishes to leave. It may well be in the patient's long-term interest to escape a medical history which includes reference to compulsory detention—particularly if this is the first presentation of mental illness. The realities of practice are that the sometimes dismal surroundings of old psychiatric hospitals, and the presence of other disturbed patients, may mitigate against an earlier genuine intent to stay in hospital, but the clinician will have in mind the possibility of the patient developing a relationship with staff and benefiting from treatment so that informal status may be maintained.

The law is inevitably insensitive to the needs of the individual and should be interpreted to achieve the optimum clinical and personal benefit to each patient.

*SECTION 5(4): NURSES' HOLDING POWER*

This section enables a nurse of a prescribed class (trained in nursing people suffering from mental illness or mental handicap (impairment) to detain an informal patient already being treated for mental disorder, for up to six hours, if conditions 2 and 3 for compulsory detention are met (p. 225), if it is not practicable to secure the immediate attendance of a medical practitioner for the purpose of a report under Section 5(2).

This section ends either on the arrival of the doctor or after the six hour period. Two forms (13 and 16) have to be signed and delivered to the hospital managers. It is not a power to be used for the convenience of medical staff to postpone a need to attend the patient.

## SECTION 2: ADMISSION FOR ASSESSMENT (OR FOR ASSESSMENT FOLLOWED BY MEDICAL TREATMENT)

Lasts up to 28 days. Application may be made by the nearest relative or an approved social worker. This must be supported by two medical recommendations (one from an 'approved doctor'). The patient has the right to apply to a Mental Health Review Tribunal within 14 days of admission. The nearest relative, the managers of the hospital or the responsible medical officer (RMO) can discharge the patient —although the RMO can prevent discharge by the nearest relative.

Psychiatrists' powers under the Act are the same (and no more) as those of any other medical practitioner. A psychiatrist (MRCPsych or equivalent) or sometimes a general practitioner by virtue of special experience may be an 'approved' doctor and provide the required second recommendation. It is preferable if at least one of the medical recommendations comes from a doctor who has previous knowledge of the patient. It is usually desirable to involve an approved social worker rather than the nearest relative for two reasons. First, an additional element of objectivity can be introduced and secondly possible later recrimination can be reduced, with benefit both to the patient and the relatives. The social worker should discuss the proposed application with the nearest available relative, if possible.

TIME LIMITS FOR RECOMMENDATION AND APPLICATION

1. The applicant must have seen the patient within 14 days.
2. The doctors' examinations of the patient must be not more than five days apart.

3. The dates of the doctors' signatures must not be later than the date of application.
4. Admission must be within 14 days of the later medical recommendation.

## SECTION 4: ADMISSION FOR ASSESSMENT IN CASES OF EMERGENCY

Lasts 72 hours. Application may be made by the nearest relative or an approved social worker supported by recommedation from one doctor, preferably by one acquainted with the patient. The application states that it is of urgent necessity to admit the patient and that admission under Section 2 would involve undesirable delay. If a doctor unknown to the patient is making the recommendation, a statement as to why it was not possible to obtain a recommendation from a doctor who does know the patient has to be made.

### TIME LIMIT FOR RECOMMENDATION AND APPLICATION

The time at which the applicant (relative or social worker) last saw the patient must be within the period 24 hours ending with the time of application. The patient must be admitted within 24 hours of the medical recommendation and the second recommendation (implementing Section 2 or 3) must be within 72 hours of admission.

## SECTION 136: PERSONS IN PUBLIC PLACES

Lasts 72 hours. Allows a police officer to remove a person who appears to suffer from mental disorder in a place to which the public has access (not therefore a person's home) to a place of safety. There is a reasonable obligation on the part of the police to remain with the patient until an adequate assessment can be made and to provide details of the reasons for implementing this section. Preferably the case should be discussed with the duty psychiatrist before the person is brought to the hospital (there may be no bed available, or it may be more appropriate to take the person to another hospital). The name of the police officer involved, and the name of the police station where the officer is based, are essential details. There are *NO* official 'section' papers—any arrangements for documentation are determined locally within each district.

## FURTHER POINTS

### OTHER DETAILS OF THE ACT

Although all the forms may have been signed and completed, admission has not been achieved in a formal sense until the patient has been accepted by the 'hospital managers' (in effect, usually a representative of the administration). This representative will scrutinise the applications and recommendations for faults that may invalidate the application completely or partially—in the latter case allowing rectification within 14 days by the person who signed the faulty form. In the event of the application being completely invalid a second (new) application would have to be made, or if the patient had been admitted a Section 5(2) could be invoked by the RMO.

There are many other details connected with the Act but it is largely the responsibility of the administration to know the answers to specific technical questions. A summary of the main features of the Act has been published by the DHSS (not recommended for non-psychiatrists) and by the Royal College of Psychiatrists.

## IMPLICATIONS OF COMPULSORY DETENTION

It is a decision with serious implications to detain someone against their will and those professionally involved have a clear duty to ensure that an adequate history and examination have been taken and alternative management considered. Section 139 of the Act gives protection against litigation to persons acting in pursuance of the Act so long as the act in question was not done in bad faith or without reasonable care (to the extent that negligence was present). Proceedings must be brought by or with the consent of the Director of Public Prosecutions; the protection afforded to staff under the 1983 Act is much less than that accorded to them under the 1959 Act.

The only immediate practical consequence of implementing a Section for compulsory admission is that the police may be asked to return the patient should he leave the hospital, or assist in the original transfer to hospital. Remembering this, and also that the process of implementing the required Section takes time, can provide some protection against undue pressure to 'Section this patient' originating in anxious and perhaps less experienced personnel. No additional resources are provided to physically restrain the patient, and hospitals are not equipped to deal with potentially violent or dangerous individuals. The legal basis for giving sedating medication if appropriate (*see* Chapter 3) in an emergency and against the patient's wishes is the same whether or not a patient is held under the Act.

It is rarely necessary to invoke the Mental Health Act to obtain admission in cases of self-injury or self-poisoning and it is certainly preferable to obtain the opinion of the duty psychiatrist before steps are taken to compulsorily detain a patient.

Copies of the most commonly used forms for implementing the provisions of the Mental Health Act 1983 are contained in Appendix 2.

## INFORMAL OR COMPULSORY ADMISSION AND THE ROLE OF PERSUASION

In mental disorder where the examining doctor recommends that a patient enters hospital, this will in most cases involve the patient's agreeing to be admitted informally. If the patient is initially unwilling to enter hospital informally further explanation and exploration of the reasons for his attitude may result in agreement to informal admission. If the patient remains unconvinced is it reasonable practice to warn him that there is sufficient concern about his mental state or behaviour to recommend compulsory admission? Direct warnings are accepted (and common) practice within medicine—for example, of the dangers of smoking. Warning that failure to accept advice or treatment may lead to harmful consequences is not unethical. Informing the patient that if he does not agree to informal admission he is risking compulsory admission is clearly a different situation, but it is difficult to argue that he should not be made aware of the way the doctor is thinking—*even if* this is perceived as coercive.

From an ethical point of view the important issue is the manner in which the information is provided. If all reasonable steps have been taken to persuade the patient to agree to informal admission then a simple factual account of the doctor's judgement of the seriousness of the problem, the potential risks if admission and treatment are not accepted and the action (for compulsory admission) likely to be recommended is, in the authors' view, good practice. The fundamental protection contained within the Mental Health Acts is the patients ability to achieve *informal* admission for the treatment of mental disorder.

# 21. Consent to treatment and failure to cooperate with treatment

This chapter is concerned with issues relating to consent to treatment in general medicine and surgery as well as in psychiatry.

## CONSENT

It is unusual for patients to refuse simple forms of treatment for which they have sought medical help. It is implicit in the doctor–patient relationship that treatment is suggested for the benefit of the patient, and various codes for the guidance of doctors have been devised (*see*, for example, Bloch and Chodoff, 1981). Even the simplest treatment may involve risk of harm—accidental, or arising from complications or side-effects of the treatment. Where treatment is complex, where the outcome is uncertain, or where there is a risk (even if small) of severe, irreversible damage (e.g. some operations involving the spinal cord) the question of how much information should be volunteered (or revealed, if asked) is a matter of clinical judgement tempered by law.

'The doctrine of informed consent forms no part of English law' (BMJ Legal Correspondent, 1983) is still true as a statement at the time of publication of this book, and a moment's thought will demonstrate how difficult it is to define 'informed consent'. Information may also be a deterrent in accepting treatment. However, if 'consent' is to have meaning, some understanding of the consequences of proposed medical evaluation and treatment must be present; this presupposes adequate levels of consciousness, mental competence, and sufficient information.

## INFORMATION

Present obligations for doctors suggesting treatment have been detailed in the following way (slightly abbreviated from Paxon, 1985):

1. The doctor has a duty to warn his patient of any material risk inherent in the treatment proposed which might weigh with the patient in giving or withholding consent and to answer questions truthfully and fully.
2. Even if there is a material risk, the doctor would not be liable if he reasonably took the view that the warning would be detrimental to the patient's health by deterring him or worrying him unnecessarily.
3. What is 'material', and whether it is reasonable to withhold the warning, are matters of medical evidence to be evaluated by the court.

In other words, the doctor must make the decision on the amount of information to be revealed after full consideration of the implications for the patient.

It is prudent therefore to pay attention to (a) case law summarized annually in medical defence societies' literature, (b) medico-legal commentaries in the medical journals, (c) seek advice from medical defence societies if in doubt, and (d) discuss any dilemma with colleagues.

A standard consent form is sparse evidence that the above points have been covered and a brief note on specific issues discussed is increasingly advisable from a legal point of view.

## CONSCIOUSNESS

Treatment of the unconscious patient is the most obvious instance of treatment without consent. In an emergency this treatment may lawfully be given where it would be considered unreasonable not to treat given the particular competence of the doctor; resuscitation following cardiac arrest would be an example.

Where a patient is simply drowsy or displays a reduced level of consciousness, mental competence, as defined below, can be determined.

## MENTAL COMPETENCE

Quite simple tests (analogous to those necessary to establish competence to make a will) can be employed:

1. Can the patient give a simple description of the nature of his illness?
2. Can he describe the treatment proposed and the possible benefits and hazards?
3. Can the patient describe the consequences of not having treatment?

## MENTAL COMPETENCE WITH CO-EXISTING MENTAL DISORDER

It is evident that someone who suffers from mental disorder (as defined in ICD-9 or DSM-III) can be competent in the sense defined above in the discussion of a surgical or general medical condition but that the patient's consent or refusal may be influenced by his mental state. If applied to the patient's understanding of a mental disorder then again the above test of mental competence may be fulfilled. Under certain conditions, where the patient is considered to require treatment in hospital for the mental illness but refuses to enter the hospital as an informal patient, compulsory admission, detention and treatment may be imposed by law (*see* Chapter 20). However, treatment for illness other than mental illness cannot be imposed on the patient without consent unless the physical illness is causing the mental illness (e.g. confusion arising from pneumonia in an elderly patient), or the situation could be considered a medical emergency.

It will be immediately apparent that treatment is often given in medical practice without fulfilling the requirements of mental competence—for example, medication used to calm agitation in dementia—and that the Mental Health Act is not in fact invoked to treat patients with delirium arising from pneumonia. These present anomalies exist largely because of political and social influences on the practice of medicine relating to the concepts of the right to receive treatment and the right to refuse treatment, particularly in the realm of formal psychiatric evaluation and treatment.

Given that the practice of medicine is deemed to be for the benefit of the potential patient, a measure of protection is afforded to both those individuals who consent to treatment and those who decline or withdraw from treatment by:

1.  the professional behaviour of the doctor as guided by the profession's own disciplinary, ethical and monitoring functions;
2.  the law.

## FAILURE TO COOPERATE WITH TREATMENT
(where immediate emergency treatment is not indicated)

If it is necessary for the benefit of the patient either in relieving distress or to prevent further harm that he receive medical treatment there is an obligation to try and achieve the acceptance of this treatment. It is enough that all 'reasonable' measures are taken. ('Reasonable' will ultimately be defined by the opinion of peers—therefore do not hesitate to obtain the opinion of colleagues if your own efforts are failing to achieve cooperation.)

The patient's failure to cooperate should be reviewed under the headings relevant to consent (to treatment). If the patient is not mentally competent relatives and those who are looking after the patient should be consulted and the proper course of action agreed. Where the patient refuses treatment but is competent as defined, it is worth discussing the rationale for treatment again with the patient, in the presence of a relative (if the patient agrees to this). An example would be the refusal to accept treatment with methionine after taking an overdose of paracetamol, or a refusal to accept the gastric lavage.

Failure to cooperate with treatment may reflect unexpressed anxieties over the procedure, or an attitude arising from low self-esteem and depression ('It's pointless having any treatment when everything's so hopeless'), or simply be another conflict with authority in a disturbed adolescent. Suspicion and anger may arise in personalities characterized by aloofness, isolation and sensitivity or traits of dependency. So-called 'rational' refusal of treatment can arise from the unconscious need to deny the severity of the illness and it is important to be aware of and seek for hidden reasons for the patient's attitude. Sometimes moral or religious beliefs conflict with medical treatment. It may be helpful, if the patient agrees, to speak with an appropriate minister or religious leader, or to arrange for the patient to do so. It is possible that the patient is misinterpreting some particular tradition or dogma and discussion with the minister may produce compliance. The basic rules for dealing with the non-compliant patient are essentially those desirable when in contact with any patient:

1. *Listen*—there may be legitimate worries or concern about earlier treatment or staff attitudes.
2. *Believe* the patient.
3. *Provide information*—for most people hospitals provoke anxiety so that concentration is impaired and even careful explanation may not be absorbed on the first occasion. Consider reasonable concerns—pain, sickness, and give reassurance where possible.
4. *Allow time* for reflection, or discussion with friends or relatives. Arrange to come back to talk about any decision later or the next day.

5. *Arrange to see the patient again* if treatment is not accepted and discuss the situation with the general practitioner.
6. *Avoid rejection*—be sensitive to the fact that in a busy A & E department this can be an understandable reaction or defence (q.v.) in less experienced staff.

## DISCHARGE AGAINST MEDICAL ADVICE

It is common practice for patients taking their own discharge against advice to be presented with forms to sign accepting responsibility for the decision. These forms cannot absolve the staff from the responsibility to assess properly the patient before allowing him to leave. Again, the criterion is one of 'reasonable' steps to achieve this assessment.

The danger of the use of these forms is that they may be presented in a confronting and non-constructive manner and it is probably more satisfactory to record the details of the discharge in the medical notes or Cardex, although some staff are likely to feel less secure with this practice.

## VOLUNTARY AND SELF-HELP ORGANISATIONS

Hospital notice boards and waiting rooms in GP surgeries may advertise self-help groups or voluntary organisations for a variety of conditions or misfortunes. The number of these has increased rapidly over the past 10 to 15 years. The principles behind their formation can be sound but in most instances there is a lack of published validation of their effectiveness. In addition, the expertise of those offering guidance is likely to be very variable and some of those initiating such schemes may be unsuited for reasons of temperament or by lack of appropriate skills. In the interests of patients it would seem prudent only to defer to those organisations which are known personally or which have links with appropriate professionals known to you in the particular field.

# Appendix 1
# Assessing the psychiatric patient

*1. PRESENTING COMPLAINT*

If, in the early stages of an interview, it is impossible to begin to answer the following basic questions then another approach should be tried, for example interviewing another informant.

   a. What is the presenting complaint from the patient's point of view? The patient's own words should be used, quoting verbatim wherever possible. If an informant is used their name and relationship to the patient must be recorded.
   b. How has the problem arisen? The onset of the problem should be defined, along with a description of the course and severity of the symptoms; the effect on the patient and significant others; the success or otherwise of the patient's attempts to alleviate symptoms.
   c. What is different or worse about the problem? Why is the patient presenting here and now? What does he want from the emergency service?
   d. Has the problem occurred before? If so, where, when and how often has it occurred?
   e. How does the presenting problem relate to stresses in the patient's life? Loss and bereavement, family, work, friends, money, housing, etc.
   f. Is the patient currently under psychiatric care? If so, with whom and what are the follow-up arrangements? All current medication and psychoactive drug use should be recorded (including proprietary drugs, illegal drugs and alcohol).

g. Specific symptoms supporting probable diagnoses should be asked about directly (vegetative symptoms in depression, autonomic symptoms of anxiety, etc.).

## 2. PAST HISTORY

An understanding of the personal and medical context of a patient's symptoms is essential for effective diagnosis and treatment, so even under pressure of time it is essential to ask about:

a. *Psychiatric history.* Previous illness episodes must be defined, with their symptoms, precipitants and natural history. Past treatments including medication, ECT and periods of in-patient care must be recorded, with the patient's response to treatment.

b. *Medical history,* including current and past illnesses, treatments, hospitalizations, operations and injuries.

c. *Family psychiatric history.* Any history of alcoholism, depression, psychosis or other mental illness in family members should be obtained.

d. *Personal history.* This can be covered fairly quickly, but should include as a minimum a description of early life, family structure and the pattern of family relationships, education and work, friendships and relationships and a sexual history. Enduring lifelong patterns of mal-adaptive behaviour, or recent changes in personality or behaviour should be especially noted.

## ELICITING AND RECORDING THE MENTAL STATE EXAMINATION

### 1. APPEARANCE AND BEHAVIOUR

*Appearance* provides valuable clues to diagnosis, for example colourful bizarre dress in a manic patient or the melancholy expression of a depressed patient. Appearance should be described in everyday language and the description should include an account of the patient's dress and grooming, the amount of eye contact and any unusual or idiosyncratic features of dress, posture of movement.

The description of *behaviour* should include the patient's general attitude and cooperation as well as motor activity. The level of motor activity should be assessed (including psychomotor retardation or agitation), as should dystonic movements, tremors, posturing gestures and tics. Possible attitudes (expressed in gesture, facial expression or speech) include cooperative, aloof, guarded, overly dramatic. Phrases such as 'attention seeking' or 'manipulative', while in common use, have little value except as terms of abuse and prejudge the patient by ascribing motives for their behaviour, thus undermining the objective nature of the mental status examination. It is better to give an accurate description of the behaviour observed and discuss its causes elsewhere. Any account of behaviour should give an indication of the interviewer's rapport with the patient.

## 2. SPEECH AND LANGUAGE

Observation of the patient's *speech* can help distinguish organic from functional disorders and also help distinguish different psychiatric disorders. It should be assessed by listening to the patient's spontaneous speech or the answers to open-ended questions.

Speech is characterized by its rate, volume, form and quality. Content of speech is usually recorded under other headings such as mood, thought or perception. The rate of speech may be excessively rapid or unusually slow. Rapid speech can be distinguished from pressure of speech which represents a difficulty interrupting the patient's flow. There may be abnormalities or variations in the volume or intensity of speech, which could be loud, pressured, explosive, monotonous or lacking spontaneity. The form of speech includes vague, digressive, circumstantial speech, or brief, uninformative replies. Quality of speech includes such features as the use of jargon, speech defects, enunciation, idiosyncratic use of words or neologisms. Slurring, dysarthria, aphasia, and abnormalities of inflection or rhythm may suggest organic brain lesions. There may be evidence of perseveration.

## 3. MOOD

*Mood* is usually described both in the patient's own words, (so-called 'subjective' mood) and in terms of emotions detected by the observer ('objective' mood). These are perceived through the patient's facial expression, gestures, tone of voice and emotional responsiveness. Mood may be described, to name just a few of the many available adjectives, as fearful, angry, hostile, anxious, euphoric, sad, depressed, suspicious or labile.

Comment should be made on whether the patient's emotional responses are appropriate to his situation and history, and whether they show apathy or blunting of emotional response. Blunted affect implies that the patient expresses a full range of emotion, all of low intensity, whereas flat affect describes little or no emotional expression. When mood is labile emotions are intense and change quickly and unpredictably. Inappropriate mood refers to expressions of feeling that are socially abnormal or inconsistent with subjective mood, thought content or behaviour.

## 4. THOUGHT

The patient's *thought processes* are only accessible to an observer through his words and actions, and so description of thought processes is closely related to the descriptions of talk and behaviour.

    a. The *form of thought* is normal if the patient is able to give a logical, chronological history with reasonable detail, and the flow of ideas is directed to understandable goals. If interrupted the patient should be able to pick up his train of thought. Disordered thought may be shown by:

i. *Circumstantiality*—the patient reaches the point after numerous irrelevant digressions.

ii. *Tangentiality*—the patient veers off train of thought and does not return. This may be a symptom of mania as is:

iii. *Flight of ideas*—the patient's thoughts follow in rapid succession but train can be followed by an observer, even if the overall effect is bizarre.

iv. *Loose associations*—there is little or no apparent connection between one expressed thought and the next.

v. *Clang associations*—puns, rhymes, plays on words.

Rambling or incoherent thought with loose associations suggests psychosis or delerium.

b. *Thought content* may be impoverished, or contain abnormal ideas or beliefs. Description of thought content should always include comment on the presence or otherwise of suicidal ideas or suicidal intent (q.v.). Abnormal thoughts with specific definitions include:

i. *Ideas of reference*—inappropriate beliefs that actions or comments of others refer directly to patient.

ii. *Delusions*—fixed, false beliefs that are not affected by rational evidence to the contrary. Delusions may be fragmented, isolated and bizarre or form part of a 'delusional system' of connected beliefs. They include delusions of persecution, grandeur, infidelity, control by others, and hypochondriacal delusions.

iii. *Obsessions*—intrusive, persistent thoughts or impulses which the patient recognises as irrational but which cannot be dismissed.

    iv. *Phobias*—pathological fears recognized by the patient and others as irrational. Common phobias include agoraphobia, social phobia and fears of specific objects or situations (lifts, animals, thunderstorms, etc.).

## 5. PERCEPTUAL DISTURBANCES

*Hallucinations* can occur in all sensory modalities, and are common in psychosis and organic disorders. Auditory hallucinations are encountered most often in functional disorders, whereas visual hallucinations are more common in delirium. Patients often have to be asked directly about hallucinations. Other perceptual disturbances include illusions (misinterpretations of actual sensory stimuli), depersonalization (a subjective sense of the unreality of oneself or parts of one's body) and derealization (a sense that the external world is unreal).

## 6. COGNITIVE FUNCTION

This is usually formally tested at the end of the interview, although an assessment of attention, concentration, distractibility and level of consciousness can be made during the interview. Testing may be seen as threatening or patronizing by patients, and should be introduced with an explanation of the tests and why they are being done. Each test should be introduced with a description of what is required and, if necessary, an example.

    a. *Orientation* is tested by asking the patient's name, age, date of birth; present place, address and town; the day, date and time. Orientation is usually lost for time, place, and person in that order. Subtle degrees of disorientation are shown in the loss of the ability to order a sequence of events in time (for example describing the day's events chronologically).

b. *Memory* may be affected by organic brain disorders, or by deficits in concentration and attention. Registration is tested by the ability to repeat a series of numbers, or a previously unknown name and address immediately after hearing them. Immediate recall is lost in organic brain syndromes and can be tested by asking the patient to repeat a complex sentence, or the details of a brief story. Recent memory requires cortex and limbic structures. It can be tested by asking for recall of a name and address after 5 minutes. Remote memory requires an intact association cortex. Historical information may be distorted by confabulation. Confirmation from an informant other than the patient is required.

c. *Abstract thinking* can be assessed by giving the patient proverbs to interpret. Overelaborate or circumstantial interpretations may be found in manic patients or those with obsessional personalities. Concrete interpretations (for example 'Too many cooks spoil the broth' interpreted as 'If there's too many people in the kitchen then they won't make the soup properly') may indicate brain damage, a schizophrenic defect state or low intelligence.

d. *Calculations* may be tested by asking the patient to serially subtract 7, starting from 100. Inability to calculate suggests dominant hemisphere dysfunction. The calculation should be done in less than two minutes.

e. *Tests of constructional ability* test parietal lobe dysfunction caused by focal lesions or dementias. The patient can be asked to copy designs, draw a cube or a bicycle, or put the hands on a clock face.

## 7. *JUDGEMENT AND INSIGHT*

*Judgement and insight* can be extremely difficult to assess, but are crucial in determining to what extent a patient is likely to cooperate with treatment. Judgement is a measure of the patient's ability to see the consequences of his actions. It is assessed by observation of the patient's behaviour and by asking what the patient would do if sent home or offered treatment, or in hypothetical situations. Insight refers to the patient's understanding of his illness, and may range from complete denial of any problem to intellectual and emotional understanding of the illness. Insight can sometimes be inferred from the patient's account of the problem (for example a depressed patient may insist that his pain is caused by cancer despite reassurance).

# Appendix 2

# Forms used for implementation of the Mental Health Act 1983

These forms represent a sample of those that non-psychiatrists might commonly meet in emergencies and by no means represent the complete range of those in use.

**Form 2**

# Application by an approved social worker for admission for assessment

Mental Health Act 1983
Section 2

To the Managers of

(name and address of hospital or mental nursing home)

(your full name) I

(your office address) of

hereby apply for the admission of

(full name of patient)

of

(address of patient)

for assessment in accordance with Part II of the Mental Health Act 1983.

(name of local social services authority) I am an officer of

appointed to act as an approved social worker for the purposes of the Act.

*Complete the following section if nearest relative known*

(a) To the best of my knowledge and belief

(name and address)

is the patient's nearest relative within the meaning of the Act.
OR
(b) I understand that

(name and address)

has been authorised by

delete the phrase which does not apply
    a county court
    the patient's nearest relative

to exercise the functions under the Act of the patient's nearest relative.

delete the phrase which does not apply
    I have
    I have not yet

informed that person that this application is to be made and of his power to order the discharge of the patient.

*Complete the following section if nearest relative not known*

(a) I have been unable to ascertain who is this patient's nearest relative within in meaning of the Act.

delete the phrase
which does not
apply

OR

(b) To the best of my knowledge and belief this patient has no nearest relative within the meaning of the Act.

*The following section must be completed in all cases*

(date)    I last saw the patient on [                                                                    ]

I have interviewed the patient and I am satisfied that detention in a hospital is in all the circumstances of the case the most appropriate way of providing the care and medical treatment of which the patient stands in need.

This application is founded on two medical recommendations in the prescribed form.

If neither of the medical practitioners knew the patient before making their recommendations, please explain why you could not get a recommendation from a medical practitioner who did know the patient:-

_____

_____

_____

_____

_____

_____

Signed  _____    Date  _____

Form 3

# Joint medical recommendation for admission for assessment

Mental Health Act 1983
Section 2

(full names and addresses of both medical practitioners)

We

registered medical practitioners, recommend that

(name and address of patient)

be admitted to a hospital for assessment in accordance with Part II of the Mental Health Act 1983.

(name of first practitioner)

I

(date)

last examined this patient on

*Delete if not applicable

*I had previous acquaintance with the patient before I conducted that examination.

*I have been approved by the Secretary of State under section 12 of the Act as having special experience in the diagnosis or treatment of mental disorder.

(name of second practitioner)

I

(date)

last examined this patient on

*Delete if not applicable

*I had previous acquaintance with the patient before I conducted that examination.

*I have been approved by the Secretary of State under section 12 of the Act as having special experience in the diagnosis or treatment of mental disorder.

We are of the opinion

(a) that this patient is suffering from mental disorder of a nature or degree which warrants the detention of the patient in a hospital for assessment

AND

(b) that this patient ought to be so detained
   (i) in the interests of the patient's own health or safety

   (ii) with a view to the protection of other persons
Delete (i) or (ii) unless both apply

AND

(c) that informal admission is not appropriate in the circumstances of this case for the following reasons:-

(Reasons should state why informal admission is not appropriate)

_____

_____

_____

_____

_____

_____

Signed _____   Date _____

Signed _____   Date _____

Form 6

# Emergency application by an approved social worker for admission for assessment

Mental Health Act 1983
Section 4

**This form is to be used only for an emergency application**

To the Managers of

*(name and address of hospital or mental nursing home)*

*(your full name)* I

*(your office address)* of

hereby apply for the admission of

*(full name of patient)*

*(address of patient)* of

for assessment in accordance with Part II of the Mental Health Act 1983.

I am an officer of

*(name of local social services authority)*

appointed to act as an approved social worker for the purposes of the Act.

*(date)* I last saw the patient on

*(time)* at

I have interviewed the patient and I am satisfied that detention in a hospital is in all the circumstances of the case the most appropriate way of providing the care and medical treatment of which the patient stands in need.

In my opinion it is of urgent necessity for the patient to be admitted and detained under section 2 of the Act. Compliance with the provisions of Part II of the Act relating to applications under that section would involve undesirable delay.

This application is founded on one medical recommendation in the prescribed form.

If the medical practitioner did not know the patient before making his recommendation, please explain why you could not get a recommendation from a medical practitioner who did know the patient:-

_____

_____

_____

_____

_____

_____


Signed _____   Date _____

                                           Time _____

Form 7

## Medical recommendation for emergency admission for assessment

Mental Health Act 1983
Section 4

### THIS FORM TO BE USED ONLY FOR AN EMERGENCY APPLICATION

(name and address of medical practitioner)

I [                                                                ]

[                                                                ]

a registered medical practitioner, recommend that

(full name and address of patient)

[                                                                ]

[                                                                ]

be admitted to a hospital for assessment in accordance with Part II of the Mental Health Act 1983.

(date) I last examined this patient on [                                    ]

(time) at [                                    ]

*Delete if not applicable

*I had previous acquaintance with the patient before I conducted that examination.

*I have been approved by the Secretary of State under section 12 of the Act as having special experience in the diagnosis or treatment of mental disorder.

I am of the opinion –

(a) that this patient is suffering from mental disorder of a nature or degree which warrants the patient's detention in a hospital for assessment for at least a limited period

AND

(b) that this patient ought to be so detained

Delete (i) or (ii) unless both apply

    (i) in the interests of the patient's own health or safety

    (ii) with a view to the protection of other persons

AND

(c) that informal admission is not appropriate in the circumstances of this case.

In my opinion it is of urgent necessity for the patient to be admitted and detained under section 2 of the Act. Compliance with the provisions of Part II of the Act relating to applications under that section would involve undesirable delay.

In my opinion an emergency exists, because I estimate that compliance with those provisions would cause about [          ] hours' delay, and I consider such a delay might result in harm as follows

(state reasons)  _____

_____

_____

_____

_____

_____

to

*Delete if not applicable

*(a) the patient
*(b) those now caring for him
*(c) other persons.

I understand that the managers of the hospital to which the patient is admitted may ask me for further information relevant to this recommendation.

I was first made aware that his condition was causing anxiety, such that it might warrant immediate admission to hospital –

†Delete whichever do not apply

†(a) Today at (time) [                              ]
†(b) Yesterday
†(c) On (date if within one week) [                              ]
†(d) more than a week ago

Signed _____     Date _____

Time _____

# Report on hospital in-patient

Form 12

Mental Health Act 1983
Section 5 (2)

*(name of hospital or mental nursing home in which the patient is)*

To the Managers of

I [                                                              ] am

delete the phrase which does not apply

the registered medical practitioner

the nominee of the registered medical practitioner

in charge of the treatment of

*(full name of patient)*

who is an in-patient in this hospital and not at present liable to be detained under the Mental Health Act 1983. I hereby report, for the purposes of section 5(2) of the Act, that it appears to me that an application ought to be made under Part II of the Act for this patient's admission to hospital for the following reasons:-

(Reasons should indicate why informal treatment is no longer appropriate)

_____

_____

_____

_____

_____

_____

Signed  _____    Date  _____

Time  _____

# Suggested further reading

*PREFACE*

Murphy, G. E., and Guze, S. B. (1960): Setting limits: The management of the manipulative patient. *Am. J. Psychother.* **14,** 30–47.

*GENERAL*

American Psychiatric Association (1980): *Diagnostic and Statistical Manual of Mental Disorders* (3rd edition). Washington: American Psychiatric Association.

*Handbook of Psychiatry* (5 vols), Cambridge University Press.

Vol. 1 General Psychopathology, ed. M. Shepherd & O. L. Zangwill.

Vol. 2 Mental Disorders and Somatic Illness, ed. M. H. Lader.

Vol. 3 Psychoses of Uncertain Aetiology, ed. J. K. & L. Wing.

Vol. 4 The Neuroses and the Personality Disorders, ed. G. F. M. Russell and L. A. Hersov.

Vol. 5 The Scientific Foundations of Psychiatry, ed. M. Shepherd.

(Definitely postgraduate use only. Comprehensive, up to date. Good source book.)

Gelder, M., Gath, D. and Mayou, R. (1983): *Oxford Textbook of Psychiatry.* Oxford Med. Publications. (Most recent of major postgraduate textbooks. Very readable, common style throughout. Recommended.)

Rix, K. J. B. (ed.) (1987): *A Handbook for Trainee Psychiatrists.* London: Ballière-Tindall.

Goldberg, D. P., Benjamin, S. and Creed, F. (1986): *Psychiatry in Medical Practice.* London: Tavistock. (Undergraduate text based on Manchester psychiatry course. Emphasis is on psychiatry as a branch of medicine. Good basic book. Recommended.)

Rund, D. A. & Hutzler, J. C. (1983) *Emergency Psychiatry*. Toronto: C. V. Mosby Co.

*CHAPTER 1: APPROACHES TO PSYCHIATRIC ILLNESS*

Farrell, B. A. (1979): Mental illness: a conceptual analysis. *Psychol. Med.* **9**, 21–35.

Frank, J. D. (1979): What is psychotherapy? In: Bloch, S. (ed.): *An Introduction to the Psychotherapies*. Oxford University Press.

Hamilton, M. (ed.) (1974): *Fish's Clinical Psychopathology*. Bristol: Wright.

Kendell, R. E. (1975): *The Role of Diagnosis in Psychiatry*. Oxford: Blackwell Scientific Publications.

Wing, J. K., Cooper, J. E. and Sartorius, N. (1974): *The Present State Examination* (9th edition). Cambridge University Press.

*CHAPTER 2: EMERGENCY INTERVENTIONS*

Bancroft, J. H. J. (1979): Crisis Intervention. In: Bloch, S. (ed.): *An Introduction to the Psychotherapies*. Oxford University Press.

*CHAPTER 4: ACUTE PSYCHOSES*

Hamilton, M. (1978): Paranoid States. *Br. J. Hosp. Med.* **11**, 545–8.

Hamilton, M. (ed.) (1984): *Fish's Schizophrenia, 3rd ed.* Bristol: Wright.

Hanke, N. (1984): *Handbook of Emergency Psychiatry*. Lexington, Massachusetts: The Collamore Press.

*CHAPTER 5: PSYCHIATRIC PRESENTATIONS OF ORGANIC BRAIN DISEASE*

Lishman, W. A. (1980): *Organic Psychiatry*. Oxford: Blackwell Scientific Publications. (Definitive text and source book.)

*CHAPTER 8: PATIENTS WITH ABNORMAL PERSONALITIES*

Lewis, A. (1974): Psychopathic personality: a most elusive category. *Psychol. Med.* **4,** 133–40

Vaillant, G. E. and Perry, J. C. (1980): Personality disorders. In: Kaplan, H. I. et al. (eds): *Comprehensive Textbook of Psychiatry.* Baltimore: Williams & Wilkins.

Campbell, P. G. and Russell, G. F. M. (1983): The assessment of neurotic and personality disorders in adults. In: Russell, G. F. M. and Hersov, L. A. (eds): *Handbook of Psychiatry Vol. 4.* Cambridge University Press.

*CHAPTER 13: PSYCHIATRIC DISORDER PRESENTING WITH PHYSICAL SYMPTOMS*

Creed, F. and Pfeffer, J. M. (eds) (1982): *Medicine & Psychiatry: A Practical Approach.* London: Pitman.

Maguire, G. P. et al. (1974): Psychiatric morbidity and referral on two general medical wards. *Br. Med. J.* **1,** 268–70.

*CHAPTER 15: THE PATIENT WHO IS DYING OR SERIOUSLY ILL*

Maguire, P. (1985): Barriers to psychological care of the dying. *Br. Med. J.* **291,** 1711–13.

Parkes, C. M. (1985): Bereavement. *Br. J. Psych.* **186,** 11–17.

Parkes, C. M. (1978): Psychological reactions to the loss of a limb. In: Howells, J. G. (ed.): *Modern Perspectives in the Psychological Aspects of Surgery.* London: Macmillan.

Worden, J. W. (1984): *Grief Counselling and Grief Therapy,* pp. 53–64. London: Tavistock.

*CHAPTER 16: THE MANAGEMENT OF DELIBERATE SELF-HARM*

Hawton, K. and Catalan, J. (1985): *Attempted Suicide: A Practical Guide to its Nature and Management.* Oxford University Press.

Hawton, K. and Catalan, J. (1981): Psychiatric management of attempted suicide patients. *Br. J. Hosp. Med.* **25,** 365–372.

## CHAPTER 17: ALCOHOL AND DRUG ABUSE

Cutting, J. (1982): Neuropsychiatric consequences of alcoholism. *Br. J. Hosp. Med.* **27,** 335–42.

DHSS London (1984): *Guidelines of Good Clinical Practice in the Treatment of Drug Misuse.* London: DHSS. (Excellent brief guide.)

Edwards, G. and Gross, M. M. (1976): Alcohol dependence: provisional description of a clinical syndrome. *Br. Med. J.* **1,** 1058–61.

Rix, K. J. B. (1978): Alcohol withdrawal states. *Hosp. Update* **5,** 403–7.

Herzber, J. L. and Wolkind, S. N. (1983): Solvent sniffing in perspective. *Br. J. Hosp. Med.* **29,** 72–6.

Royal College of Psychiatrists (1986): *Alcohol: Our Favourite Drug.* Report of a Special Committee. London: Tavistock.

Sillanpaar, M. L. (1982): Alcoholism: Treatment of alcohol withdrawal symptoms. *Br. J. Hosp. Med.* **27,** 343–50.

Sourindrhin, I. (1985): Solvent misuse. *Br. Med. J.* **290,** 94–5.

## CHAPTER 18: DRUG TREATMENT OF PSYCHIATRIC EMERGENCIES

Crammer, J., Barraclough, B. and Heine, B. (1982): *The Use of Drugs in Psychiatry* (2nd ed). London: Gaskell.

Pullen, G. P., Best, N. R. and Maguire, J. (1984): Anticholinergic drug abuse: a common problem? *Br. Med. J.* **289,** 912–13.

## CHAPTER 19: DRUGS THAT MAY CAUSE PSYCHIATRIC SYMPTOMS

King, D. J. (1986): Drug induced psychiatric syndromes. *Prescribers' Journal* **26,** 50–8.

*CHAPTER 20: MENTAL ILLNESS AND THE LAW*
DHSS (1983): *Mental Health Act (1983): Memorandum on parts I-VI, VIII & X.* London: DHSS.
Royal College of Psychiatrists (1983): *The Mental Health Act (1983): Summary of Main Provisions.* London: Royal College of Psychiatrists. (Two booklets; one relating to England and Wales, one to Scotland.)

*CHAPTER 21: CONSENT TO TREATMENT AND FAILURE TO COOPERATE WITH TREATMENT*
Appelbaum, P., Roth, S. and Loren, H. (1984): Involuntary treatment in medicine and psychiatry. *Am. J. Psychiat.* **141,** 202–5.
Bloch, S., and Chodoff, P. (1981): *Psychiatric Ethics,* Appendix. Oxford University Press.
BMJ Legal Correspondent (1983): Treatment without consent; emergency. *Br. Med. J.* **290,** 1505–6.
Puxon, M., (1985): Informed consent. *Br. J. Hosp. Med.* **33,** 6.
Editorial (1980): In search of true freedom: Drug refusal, involuntary medication and 'Rotting with your rights on'. *Am. J. Psychiat.* **137,** 327–8.

# Glossary of psychiatric terms
(Modified from the *Manchester Handbook of Psychiatry for Medical Students.*)

*Affect.* The patient's emotional state judged subjectively by the recognition of emotions in oneself and objectively (by facial expression, posture, etc.) in others. *Lability* of affect. When mood fluctuates rapidly from one state to another. *Blunting* of affect. Constriction of the range of normal emotional responsiveness.

*Agitation.* Increased motor activity associated with marked anxiety; includes fidgeting, restlessness, handwringing, pacing.

*Anxiety.* Mood of fear, apprehension or a sense of danger; autonomic symptoms (q.v.) may be present. *Free-floating* anxiety. Persistent anxious mood in the absence of provoking circumstances. *Phobic* anxiety. Anxiety provoked (irrationally) by specific situations, such as crowds, confinement, animals. These situations are usually avoided.

*Automatism.* A simple or complex motor act carried out with apparent unawareness of the environment.

*Catastrophic reaction.* An explosive expression of affect which occurs when a patient attempts a task beyond his capabilities.

*Catatonia.* A variety of motor behaviours including automatic obedience, negativism, posturing and waxy flexibility.

*Circumstantiality.* Long-winded, pedantic speech with many unnecessary details, although remaining goal-directed.

*Clouding of consciousness.* Diminution of the level of consciousness; evidenced by reduced and fluctuating awareness of the environment, diminished grasp and drowsiness.

*Compulsive acts.* Acts which are experienced as having to be carried out (to prevent anxiety) despite attempts to resist and the knowledge that the act is irrational.

*Confabulation.* Changing, loosely held and falsified memories which conceal an amnesia of organic origin.

*Delirium.* Clouding of consciousness associated with hallucinations and psychomotor agitation.

*Delusion.* False belief held with total conviction and inappropriate to the patient's intelligence, social background and culture beliefs. It is the intensity with which the belief is held rather than its falseness which is the main morbid feature.

*Depression.* A mood of sadness, misery or dejection. When associated with other symptoms (q.v.) may become morbid.

*Elation* (also *euphoria*). State of well-being, optimism, cheerfulness which may be morbid when out of keeping with the situation.

*Flight of ideas.* A disorder of thought, manifested in speech, in which the patient wanders from one theme to another on the basis of a variety of verbal associations or distracting stimuli. The tempo of speech may be increased.

*Fugue.* A sudden disturbance of behaviour characterised by wandering, associated with subsequent partial or total amnesia.

*Hallucination.* A false sensory perception lacking an adequate basis in external reality.

*Hypochondriasis.* An abnormal preoccupation with real, imagined or anticipated ill-health.

*Ideas of reference.* The idea that an event refers specially to the patient when in reality it has no such significance.

*Illusion.* A false perception based on the misinterpretation of a real stimulus.

*Neologism.* A new word specially constructed by the patient which may form part of a private language.

*Obsession.* An unpleasant thought, causing great anxiety, which intrudes into consciousness in spite of attempts to resist it and which is recognised as irrational.

*Panic attack.* A discrete episode of intense fear and anxiety, with autonomic accompaniments, which the patient seeks to end by urgent avoiding action.

*Passivity.* The false belief that the patient is passively and unwillingly controlled by an alien force which penetrates his mind or body.

*Perseveration.* The persistence of a verbal or motor response after it has ceased to be appropriate.

*Phobia.* A fear which is out of proportion to the stimulus, cannot be explained or reasoned away and leads to avoidance of the feared situation.

*Pressure of speech.* Speech that is excessive in speed, quantity or both.

*Pseudohallucination.* A form of hallucination characterised by the experience of a false percept in inner subjective space (e.g. voices 'inside my head') and lacking the vividness and depth of a true hallucination. It may have an 'as if' quality ('I saw him just as if he was still alive').

*Retardation.* The morbid slowing of thought or movement.

*Stereotypies.* Utterances or movements which are monotonously repeated, non goal-directed and do not seem to have any special significance for the patient.

*Stupor.* A state of almost complete absence of movement and speech with the preservation of consciousness (inferred from appropriately directed eye movements).

*Thought block.* The sudden cessation of a train of thought resulting in a complete but brief absence of thoughts.

*Thought broadcasting.* The belief that the patient's private thoughts are being made known to and shared by others.

*Thought echo.* The experience of thoughts being repeated or echoed out loud.

*Thought insertion.* The experience of intrusion into the patient's mind of thoughts that he experiences as definitely not his own.

*Thought withdrawal.* The experience that thoughts are being removed from the patient's mind.

*Torpor.* A state of pathological drowsiness with a tendency to fall into a dreamless sleep.

*Twilight state.* In which conscious awareness is narrowed down to a few ideas and attitudes.

*Waxy flexibility.* A feeling of plastic resistance, like bending a soft wax rod, when the examiner moves the patient's body; the posture may be preserved when the passive movement stops.

# INDEX

271